From H2H to ME
Thank you For all of
your Help.

MORE
BETTER
HAPPIER

MORE
BETTER
HAPPIER

A psychologist's letter to his kids,
disguised as leadership.

dr. jason richardson

"This is one of those books you just can't put down. Disguised as a letter to his kids filled with so many AHA becomes a fun exploration and manual within a story-driven ride by embracing the three real core areas of your own life. Don't walk, run. It's that good!"

- Bryan Kramer, CEO at PureMatter & H2H Companies, Best Selling Author of books: USA Top 100 Book 'Shareology' and "Human-to-Human', TEDTalk

"More, Better, Happier is a blueprint to navigating your personal growth in today's chaotic personal, economical, political, and dynamic workplace environment.

Don't let the title fool you, MBH allows you to reflect deeply on who you are and why you think and feel the way do; then gives you the steps for the growth needed to lead a life of abundance and happiness."

- Gregg Frederick, MBA, CSE

"I believe this book is truly a snapshot of Jason's best attributes as a Psychologist, Athlete, and Entrepreneur. He has the rare ability to call you out on your limitations with wit and kindness, and help you get refocused on the right steps to help you become more, better, and happier."

- Dr. Melissa Longo

"If you want more in your life that it starts with accepting and honoring the responsibility that comes with it. Dr. Richardson demonstrates and carves a clear pathway to achieve that responsibility. This book is the manual on how to navigate the road to getting 'more, better and happier' with the simplistic way of actually needing less to getting it."

- Greg Romero

"Reading this book gave me more "aha's" than I've had in awhile! Dr. Jason offers a holistic perspective on fulfillment, and calls on authentic accountability for the life we create. This book was relatable, tangible, timely, thought provoking and offers clear strategies that can be implemented immediately to be more, better and happier!"

- Dr. Karen Quinn

"How we think about things just may be the problem! In MBH, Dr. J Rich brilliantly challenges how we think about ourselves, others and the world. Truth be told your More, Better, and Happier probably isn't as far off as you think..."

- Clarence M. Lee, Jr., M.D., MBA

Edited by:
George E. Jones, Jr.
Jim Rusnak

Table of Contents

1

Election Cycle

Your vote counts?

In eighth grade, I ran for class president. As soon as I could, I went to work on making the posters. I talked to my classmates about all the issues affecting eighth-graders and my constituency seemed to be in full support of my ideas.

"Yeah, we SHOULD do that!"

"That's a good idea."

My personal favorite, "I like your posters!"

Two other candidates were running against me: Brian and Georgiana. On the day of the election, the three of us gave our speeches before the class voted. Given my temperament—me being me—I eagerly anticipated this moment and volunteered first to address the classroom.

No talking about the other candidates. No talking about any eighth grade frivolities one could expect on after-school television or their favorite sitcom. Just serious straight-talk about what I was willing to do for my classmates. I presented arguments about how I was ready to stand up for our rights, addressed all the lunchtime and recess complaints about the small, private Catholic school we attended, and how I would bring those grievances to the teachers and principal at Assumption Memorial School. Not only did I say what I would do, I even provided examples of previous advocacy—nothing but the facts! This was the spirit of my election speech.

Next up was Georgiana. She was smart and very articulate— way more mature than all of us. She would have been my choice had I not been in the race myself. Georgianna's speech was simple and clean, a very "I will do my best to be a good president" type of message.

Then came Brian. He was the most popular, AND he was

well-liked. There is a difference between the two, especially in eighth grade. He talked about what he wasn't going to do. One of the main things he wasn't going to do was make promises he couldn't keep. Somehow, it felt like everything *he* was talking about was directed at, or against, *me*!

In my head, I was thinking:
"Why does everyone else seem to like what he is saying...?"
"But, I DID mean what I said!"
"I even gave proof during my speech..."
To top things off, he didn't even care if he won or not. He was kinda like, "I'll do it if you want me to."
"You frickin' kidding me, 'I'll do it if you want me to!?'"
"Seriously!?"
"....and why does the class seem to like this?"
What's going on?

After the speeches, the teacher gave us the instructions and voting slips. It was time to vote. I wanted to win but wasn't necessarily expecting to win. Still, there was hope.

Our teacher wrote the results on the board as a couple of classmates counted the votes:

Brian was the clear winner.

Georgianna had the remainder of the votes, with one exception.

I got one vote. The only vote I received was my own.

2

Rules for Engagement

How to read this book
(and possibly get through the rest of your life).

You make the rules, really. Honestly (and more on honesty in a few short paragraphs), you've been either consciously or unconsciously making and accepting rules your entire life. We accept societal rules, educational rules, familial rules, workplace rules, traffic rules, etc., integrating and amending specific sets of rules along the way to match up with whatever values, belief systems, or reasons you need to maintain your perceptions of order. Or keep your sanity. Or just get yourself through the day—and on *to* the next day.

Rules dictate your life, whether you think they do or not.

As a "pre-rule" of sorts, I encourage you to allow the following rules for the sake of getting through this text. They are as follows:

1. Be more open

I know! You have heard this one before. But I am saying "be MORE open…" not just (rolling my eyes) "be open." No need to change all of who you are and what you know. I would like you to leave room to integrate possible different ways to look at and do things. As soon as you take on the "I've-heard-this-before" attitude, you have closed yourself off. All of us know stuff, and yet haven't truly let what we "know" sync in a way that informs our thoughts and actions to be better. True—you may KNOW this intellectually… But do you do this? Is this knowledge incorporated in your DNA?.

You HAVE heard this before—probably because you need to listen to it. Knowing something and doing something are not the same. You know eating that bag of chips is not the right choice all the time. You know you have work to do. You know you should've gone to the gym today. You know you've been avoiding your prostate exam. You know starting your work sooner is probably better. You know making your bed and putting your clothes away IS the better course of regular daily action.

But… do you?

Being more open means accepting the possibility that what you know, who you are, and what you are capable of can grow, evolve, and progress in any direction. Saying you've "heard this before" is dismissive, not informative or constructive. Knowing is not enough. Raising consciousness sounds essential, but let's be real. It's only great if your behavior changes and is in alignment with your new awareness. And if you want to be honest, it is only great if your new understanding and behavior generally generate positive outcomes. And if you really, really want to be honest, assess whether those positive outcomes are only good for you, or if they lift you as well as others, generally.

2. Be radically honest with yourself. Brutally honest—without beating yourself up!

Our brains do a great job of explaining things, a.k.a creating excuses. This is especially true when we fall short of our expectations, or maybe do something that contradicts what we know. Factually and mathematically, there probably is a real explanation for why you keep coming up short:

Maybe they did cheat.

Maybe you made a mistake.

Maybe the boss was always going to choose his son?

Maybe you do (or don't) fit the description?

Maybe you aren't as good as you thought?

Maybe, just maybe—it's not them?

Maybe—it's not unfair?

Maybe it's not the system, racism, oppression, patriarchy, matriarchy, or the league　　　　　(little, big, pro, or otherwise), or those ridiculous HOA rules!

Maybe it's the way you think.

Maybe it's what you're doing or not doing… or not willing to do?

Maybe those explanations are excuses.

Maybe I wasn't the best person to be class president in the eigth grade?

Maybe I confused others' politeness for agreement?

Rule #2 is NOT about beating yourself up. Rule #2 is, however, about holding yourself up to a standard that is, just a bit, higher than you feel comfortable. It is a look at what you're doing, rather than what you're getting. Because it's what you do that allows you to get what you want. What's going well — and what's not going well — in your business, sport, and life? What things can you do that will probably make things better for you and those around you? What things can you give up doing that would do the same? Dig deep and get real with yourself. I trust you'll know if you're lying to yourself. Once you get to the truth, you always have the choice to step up.

One last thing about this rule — it could very well be the system, racism, oppression, patriarchy, or the league. And that, indeed, sucks. I still urge you not to let that be the reason you are not working toward more, better, and happier. You still live with you, regardless of the game you choose to play or get roped into by happenstance

.

3. Commit to step up!

We spend a lot of time avoiding things. Consciously or unconsciously. Brains are built to survive and avoid threats. While it's prudent to avoid stepping into the street before looking both ways, involving yourself in political conversation at work, or doing the same with family, I ask you to ask yourself:

- What am I, or have I been avoiding?

- What is the fear that will be validated? (Refer back to Rule #2)

To progress—not stagnate or regress—you will want to become comfortable with the fact that you may lack the skill or knowledge required to get what you want. You will want to admit that you may have lost (as in, did NOT qualify or meet the standard) more times than you've won. You will want to accept there's much more to do in your efforts to live your dream. If not, you are just living in a dream world.

If you are cool with the latter, reading this book isn't what you signed up for. If you are cool with the former, then it's time to step up to the fact that course correction, obtaining knowledge/skills, and demonstrating courage are your responsibilities.

Stepping up is about raising YOUR capacity not just to work harder, but to raise yourself to another level. There will be more on this later. Plenty of people sedate themselves with work. Plenty of people medicate themselves with busyness. Doing what is hard helps you become stronger, yes. Doing what is hard for YOU helps you become more for yourself and to others. Stepping up is taking that brutal honesty and working to apply it with consistency. Which leads directly to the next rule…

4. Make it YOURS!

I do not know everything, but I know the heck out of what I do know. There are fundamental principles that serve as a foundation for almost every business, sport, and life concept. While fundamentals are generally accepted as universal, the secret sauce is about applying who YOU ARE to those fundamentals.

We tend to think our favorite athlete has the perfect swing or throw until someone else comes along with another perfect swing or throw. You see things like "best practices," until the old best practices are updated or upended by the disruptors, influencers, and innovators. I am not saying you shouldn't study the best—I want you to study the best. It's great when we learn smart from the smart, good from the good, and right from the right. I also want you to add YOU to all of that learning. Because you are not the people you study. You are the last percentage points that make the perfect swing you learned more perfect. It's YOU who is living YOUR life, not someone else's! Incorporating your DNA into a fundamental framework is the secret. Steph Curry's jumper is HIS, and we love it—or hate it if you're not a fan! Which leads directly to the next rule…

5. Share the *WELLth. Yes, W-E-L-L-th!

Steph Curry may not share all of his success secrets on the court, but he shares that jumper with the world every time we watch him play. Either way, both he and the world are better for it by way of entertainment for the fans, a five-year, 200-million-dollar contract for him, and basketball players around the globe working to step up (remember Rule #3?) the next time they get on the court.

As it pertains to becoming more, better, and happier—for your sake and others—share as best as you can everything you glean from this book (with all due credits, of course) with family, friends, teammates, and co-workers because:

Sharing with WELLth is one way of Making it Yours, and:

The world will be better for it because you're the one doing the sharing, much like Steph Curry's jumper. But, I'm not guaranteeing you'll get a 200 million dollar contract!

6. You will be offended! And hopefully... not too triggered. Sorry—not sorry.

To get to the other side of this, you'd better want to face some of the things you've been avoiding. I am working to interrupt the thoughts, behaviors, and patterns that don't allow you to be more, better, and happier. In some of my examples, the language is not necessarily my language, but rather the language of the zeitgeist. We read it and hear it across all the channels to which we avail ourselves. It's the language that, unfortunately, people have taken too seriously AND for granted at the same time. I use it to elicit an emotional response and/or illustrate a point, while asking you (maybe even compelling you) to think independently from the conventional, the group, or the zeitgeist.

I will test your sensibilities as you move through the pages, just as they are tested in life. Please, do not let anyone stand in your way of progress—even if that person, a system, or your own hurt feelings are working to impede it.

Again... What you are about to read is an interruption of your usual patterns that will help you get to the truth. It's worth the risk of offending you—not to be rude, but to engage you in real conversations about things that matter. I do my best to take a 360 degree approach.

I want you to recognize the obvious—which is the fact that we're all here now, that we're all human, and probably want many of the same, fundamental things. Solutions on economic disparity,

racial inequities, climate change, and politics do not exist within the next few pages, but I do believe all of those things may not affect you as much if you apply what you are about to read.

No one is coming to save you.

But there are things you can do to save yourself and possibly those close to you.

By doing those things , we may just end up saving each other.

#morebetterhappier

Conflict

"Baby, it takes people a very long time to learn a very little."

James Baldwin

3

Domestic Silence

Remember the trigger warnings!

Our time, or all-time?

We live in a time where everything we want is literally at our fingertips. It's (almost) like 'The Jetsons.' You press a button; food shows up. You swipe right or left, and you have a date for the night. You click 'Buy It Now,' and whatever it was you just bought arrives at your door within 48 hours—or even on the same day! You have a question—Siri and Alexa are standing by with an answer. They will even offer other options and suggestions if you do happen to stump the internet. You can learn why using the word *'supposebly* 'is, in fact, incorrect. *Supposedly,* there's an app for that, too! And by that, I mean any THAT you conjure in your mind. Never before has it been so easy to get anything. Or maybe it's more appropriate to say, never before has it been so easy to get any one thing.

So why is it we all seem to feel like we lack so much? What's missing? And why does it seem everyone is arguing about every damn thing?

It's not the things we say, but rather the rhetoric we continue to hear from either end of the political spectrum on what seems to be every issue. It could be that it's not about voicing YOUR concern as much as it is silencing those with whom we disagree. Or, it could be you are silencing yourself for fear of ridicule from the majority. Statistically, those making the most noise are NOT in the majority, but rather on the margins. They are however, loud, organized, and funded in many cases. Either way, it has become far too easy to stand behind a fabricated line and argue with anonymity than it is to state your opinion publicly. It seems it's the things we don't say that might be getting us all in a tizzy.

The world is big—and at the same time shrinking—as we hurtle through space and scroll our way through emails, selfies, best-days-ever, tweets, snaps, and "wait for it, wait for it…. OMG—This just happened…!» The ubiquity, usage, and consumption of social media illustrate how our attention to everything has us inundated with information. Lots of information! We take in far more than we can process. Unfortunately, we think we process far more than we are taking in.

Artificial Intelligence (AI) curates what we see through complex algorithms. It selects content for you based on your behavior and preferences, and sprinkles in what's trending and who's (not) engaging. That same AI is also listening, watching, grouping, predicting, and pushing us to think and behave in specific ways. (Election, lately? It seems we are always in a constant election cycle.) Neuroscience states the majority of the thoughts you had today are the thoughts you had yesterday. Interestingly enough, your feeds mimic this as you scroll the same stories, memes, and events that support your belief systems, values, and idealized self. Often, it's a caricatured image of your self-identity.

Republican or Democrat?

"But what about the Green Party?"

Conservative or Liberal?

"But what about the alt-right and far-left?"

Are you privileged, or am I underprivileged?

"My race is supposed to tell you no to the former, but my education and bank account don't jibe with with the latter."

Vegan? Keto?

"But what happened to the food pyramid and the south beach diet?"

Traditional? Disruptive?

"But what about those who just want to do their job so they can get back home to their family?"

Is it they, or is it you? "They" being those tech giants. "They" being those greedy land developers. "They" being those snowflakes. "They" being those corrupt politicians. "They" being those one-percenters. "They" being those anti-vaxxers. "They" being those... people!

"What do you mean, 'Those people?'»

"Maybe you mean, 'You people?'»

I mean, US, people!

Maybe, just maybe...?

The stories we tell ourselves have all been told before by previous generations, but the difference is we amplify our thoughts today through 4G, LTE, and (possible cancer causing?) 5G networks. If you're reading this, you have access to a soapbox via pick-your-favorite-platform (FB, IG, Twitter, etc.). We already have a natural propensity to become drawn in by conflict and drama. Add advertisers competing for a space on our soapboxes, and we can easily see that the loudest, most controversial, or most provocative headlines (again, carefully curated for us) rise to the top of our feeds. None of us can take our eyes off the proverbial train wreck. There's an incentive to perpetuate such an environment. More conflict means more eyes on the screen, which in turn generates more dollars from advertisers. The more you stay, click, like, comment, post, share, and buy, the more data they collect from you.

Most of us are all too happy to participate. And why not? We can keep up with our family, reacquaint with a college roommate, and lurk our next potential hire, fire, or romantic interest. You're not necessarily trying to be an influencer; he's not looking to run for office; and she's not trying to be any spokesperson for a group or cause. But don't pick the "wrong" side, otherwise you will be at risk.

Plenty of good (if not good, decent) people find themselves shamed, slandered, or dismissed by those on the "right" side (irony intended) of an issue. You may find yourself choosing to silence yourself, getting silenced, or doubling down on an opinion that started as a fleeting thought or honest question. We sometimes don't make sense to ourselves when others are on the offensive.

As far as I can tell, there's a hierarchy of identifying labels as it pertains to whom to target, or whether person or group can be held accountable at all. Suppose you're in a group considered disadvantaged, and you disagree with someone on another disadvantaged side. In that case, the other disadvantaged side will leave you alone and go after the person on the most advantaged side that opposes them. Did you get that? Me neither!

An excellent example of this behavior was the Prop 8 measure on gay marriage in California back in 2008. Proponents of Prop 8 vilified white, conservative Christians for that measure not passing, but the black and hispanic vote sealed the deal. This episode demonstrated what humans have done over the course of all humanhood. That is, it's easier to go after the group that seems like it can be gone after. It's no different than in junior high. Bullies pick fights with the kids who won't fight back, or those they see as not strong enough to win   .

The prevailing wisdom is you just can't attack an already-oppressed people, regardless of which side of history they lie. Further, that wisdom tells us darker-skinned people MUST be more virtuous than their fair-skinned, European counterparts, don't they? There seems to be an unwritten and complex algorithm based on what we happen to be, versus who we are and how we act, when it comes to public opinion. We have taken the "you-can't-say-bomb-on-an-airplane!" mentality and applied it to anything remotely, indirectly, or inadvertently not part of popular opinion, in-group vernacular, or the previous generation's understanding of that they know vs. what they are supposed to know now. (Yes, Gen Y and Z. You, too, will eventually join the *'out-of-touch club'* — and probably quicker than your predecessors.) We are training ourselves to become offended. If you have no problems, you have no problem. And if you have no problem, you have no platform.

In 2021, it seems there are far more groups — with far more rules — fighting for their rights than in 2008. Or, are there just more platforms and soapboxes? Or, could it be that the better it gets for the whole, the more the whole can find discrepancies, injustices, offenses, and inconsistencies in the systems, policies, institutions, and others? The rulesets belonging to specific groups have grown exponentially in quantity and complexity. Some label others as an "ist," when in actuality, the speed of technology, coupled with the inherent gaps between generations, make it difficult for everyone to keep up. My in-laws are sweet, loving people. They also are not on Twitter, and thus not up to date on all of the new rules regarding pronouns, descriptors, and labels. As far as they are concerned, their generation was working to get rid of labels. You can see the confusion.

The reality is, many of us are at war with ourselves. Many have not made peace with their pasts. People who are not happy with where they are, what they are, or who they are, can find it easy to pick sides or to posse-up. They point the fingers at "them" and find comfort with those who share "their truth." With all the talk of of woke, hustle, 10X, resist, (insert hashtags here), we seem to forget that most of the things we find fault in are within the significant advances we all enjoy. In other words, we all have gotten so used to a standard of living — one far greater than 10, 20, or 40 years ago — that we're pointing out what's wrong with "the system" as we're lamenting the dead spot we hit while traveling through town, causing Face-Time to freeze, while listening to streamed music over Spotify as we drive our electric car to get food from the grocery store that we ordered on Instacart. Or… something like that.

For the record, I DO NOT condone racism, malicious hate, bigotry, or stacking the deck (cheating). I also recognize that your ass and mine can get shut down, fired, or raked through the mud if we misunderstand or step across the ever-growing number of lines drawn in various directions! It's far too easy for the mob to ask you (im)politely to step down for private opinions. Some of us will answer to our 17, 18, 22-year-old selves at the age of 45, 55, and 60. I mean, really, y'all should've had it all figured out by the age of 16, right?!? And yes, we are well-served to figure it out — but that takes a lifetime.

Is it good policy to judge history through the lens of current events, our truths (or your truths), and the zeitgeist of the last 10 years, 5 years, or... year? The people on the "right side" of history want to take away your platform based on your imperfect past. How can clairvoyance be a prerequisite for well-adapted behavior in society?

Never mind the fact that you were a dumb kid just trying to fit in.

Never mind the fact that none of us know what we don't know.

Never mind the fact that your opinions have changed — or that you have learned and grown.

Never mind the fact that those pointing the finger at you probably — definitely — have their own cringeworthy, embarrassing, and shameful moments in their past. Again, this is not about excusing bad behavior. We keep convicted murderers, rapists, and pedophiles away from society for good reasons.

__Before we go further…

Pause.

Breathe… in through the nose and out through the mouth.

———

Remember rule #6? If not, refer to rule #6 again. If so, please know I am not excusing rapists from rape or murderers from murder. Both clinically and personally, my experience is people do things that do not even make sense to themselves. For example, you might hold the belief that you are an honest person, but you lie to your spouse about how much you spent on the new toy in the garage. You know… the vegetarian who only eats meat on holidays, Sundays, and when "their body needs it?!?" All jabs aside, some people's opinions *do* change over time. What they value can change over time. My points above have more to do with getting fired at the age of 50 for something you said in private when you were 20. No one's thoughts are entirely pure (if you want to push back on that, I would suggest you do research on the MMPI). No one's track-record is free of blemishes. We shouldn't just think about the skeletons hidden in our closets, but the ones we forgot about when we moved to the new house. That goes for the finger pointers as well as the ones accused.

We publicly, and (anti)socially, battle issues as if the world is coming to an end tomorrow. There is no bomb on the airplane. At least not all of them! The world has been coming to an end ever since I can remember my parents watching the news in our linoleum-floored, Formica-countertopped kitchen back in the '80s. The same cast of characters, too! Russia vs. the USA, turmoil in the Middle East, the Republican guy (pretty much any of them) telling you he will lower taxes, the Democrat person (pretty much any of them) telling you they will provide more programs.

Fast forward to the '08, '12, '16, and 2020 US elections — we went from a black (or African-American) President telling us America is still racist, to a billionaire President telling us he is "just like you." I over simplify the message, but that is the point. Was that their message? Or was that what we construed from the messaging? Regardless of which party was in charge, we went to war with other countries (the ones we know have no real power), on ideologies, drugs, inanimate objects, and, unfortunately, each other. While I'm up for a good fight as much as anyone, I am not sure all of the battles we pick are worth the energy we spend and punches we throw. Though some fights sure get us going and make for a good headline. But, who are we fighting anyway?

Aren't we related to some of those people?

Don't we live with those people?

Isn't it possible we love some of those people?

Maybe some of those deplorables and libtards (not my words!) are in your family.

Perhaps that deplorable held the door open for you.

Maybe that libtard helped you close a deal or hit a sales goal.

Maybe the disadvantaged and oppressed are not as pious as you might think, or as disadvantaged or oppressed as you thought.

Maybe that person with privilege is suffering in ways you do not see — or value.

Perhaps, we might get along with that deplorable or libtard if we didn't know their politics, diet concerns, or choice of partner? Or once you realize you both like to drink, smoke, and go fishing.

Maybe we like them only because we know these things?

Maybe some of us fell in love with a libtard.

Maybe we didn't know they were deplorable until we saw their last Facebook post?

Maybe they're not deplorable, just insensitive, or unaware.

Perhaps the libtard just disagrees with your worldview and wants to see people get a fair shake?

How can it be that half a country is reprehensible and the

other half is intellectually disabled? (The editor told me not to use the word libtard). Aren't some of those intellectually disabled our neighbors? Don't we work with some of those racists? Real question is, if someone can be racist and still work with you or hire you, aren't they, at the very least, putting *their* issues aside? They not liking you, but dealing with you, is tolerance. A low bar, yes. But if they can get over their stuff to get the job done, shouldn't we all get over OUR stuff… just a bit? Have you liked (or even respected) every person you've ever worked with?

Enter, Donald Sterling, owner of the Los Angeles Clippers basketball team, banned for life from the NBA in 2014 for making racist remarks. Ironically, this guy paid out millions to the very people whom he so despised, inadvertently contributing to the resources and platforms of said despised people to act on any causes they deem important—racism included. Unlike the 1600s, 1700s, 1800s, and a good portion of the 1900s, no one was forcing anyone to take the money, play for that team, or anything else. I would respect a player who declines to work for such a person. I'm also not hating on any player for getting out on the court. Keep in mind, I am sure the coaches and players didn't know these things about

the team owner before they signed. Alas, it was his biracial girl-friend who outed him vis á vis an undisclosed recorded conversa-tion. For the record, we DON'T need people like that in the NBA or any organization. I do, however, want us to be able to look at these things from all angles.

While it's preferable to be liked, respected, and hired, it's like-ly the case we sometimes won't get all three at our place of employ, in the world, or even in our own families, despite our best efforts. It is nice when it happens, and it happens well inside the bell of the bell curve! Unfortunately, things going along swimmingly are not headline material.

Your co-worker wants what's best for her family, too. Your spouse, most likely, doesn't want to disappoint you. The people in your family might belong to a union, and the family you married into might be a bunch business owners or "corporate-types." The old white male might be a tremendous ally. Your friend who smokes too much weed didn't get the job because he smokes too much weed—not because he is black or gay. Or maybe they got the job because they are black and gay?! I've seen it happen. I used to work in social services.

———

Before we go further…

Pause.

Breathe… in through the nose and out through the mouth.

Remember I said you would get offended? If not, refer to rule #6 again!

———

If we're being brutally honest, it isn't fair that people overlook behavior in some groups and frown upon in others. I can say the "N-word," and some of you can't—or better not! And let's be real, women are just as capable of leaving the toilet seat up just as much as men are at leaving it down. If you want to go about changing such injustices—whether toilet seats or racism—fine. However, make sure you're holding yourself up to the same standard as the institutions you want to change.

If you think I just trivialized racism by comparing it to leaving the toilet seat up—well, despite popular opinion, I am black and asian (or middle-eastern depending on perspective). I've experienced discrimination and disappointed my wife. Both are personal. Both hurt. We're all independent agents acting on sets of values, experiences, and information—just trying to get through our respective lives the best we can. Some actions have considerably more consequences than others, but from a human behavior perspective—from a reduced-to-absurdity standpoint—we are all guilty of not making sense as we rail at the world and others for not making sense. All of us have done things that don't make sense. I'm asking you to make sense of your own behavior first. If we do this, we might be too busy improving ourselves to worry about fixing others. By the way, you are not broke(n), even if it feels that way.

Yes, I realize the irony of me talking about our irony. Alas, irony seems to be a built-in feature of the human experience. There'll be more on that later.

A black man becoming president of the United States is amazing, especially given what we know about the history of the United States. The billionaire, any billionaire, running for office IS no different than you. Not all wealth is inherited. Not all privilege is financially, racially, or gender-based. Keep in mind, Obama's children are now privileged. LeBron James' kids are now privileged. Also keep in mind, if one doesn't know who those kids are, what identity do you think most others would ascribe to those children? A black person shouldn't have to become a president or the best basketball player in the world for their children to be treated fairly. I suppose the children of celebrity and political figures, if one knows who they are, wouldn't be treated fairly or equally. I will let you decide whether that treatment is just or unjust—right or wrong. We also can't deny that while there are disparities as it relates to socio-economic status, there is a Congressional Black Caucus, there was a two-term African-American president, and as this is being written, a female vice-president of back and asian decent. Somehow, they got there. My guess is that it was hard fought, well-earned, and with the help of many people who identify in many different ways with different individual tastes, agendas, and looks.

For every Trump, there is a Warren Buffett. For every Obama, there is a Sharpton. You can choose who you'd like at your dinner table. But be clear about this: you have the capability of either party, or group, or cause (pun intended) at either end of the continuum. Both you and I are just as capable of what's good and right as much as we are what's dishonorable and deceitful. The degree to which we behave in those ways varies based on our beliefs and perceptions of the world, ourselves, and others. And, of course, the fact that our brains will always justify our own behavior. Recognize, they (whichever "they" you choose) may not be against you as much as they are for them. You may want to ask yourself before you decide to fight, "Am I fighting for, with, or against?"

Somebody is going to win, and it may as well be you. Everyone will experience loss, and while I wish the best for everyone, it's the case that losing happens anyway. The question is, can you string together enough wins over all the periods in your life? Can you learn from your losses, even though life is, in fact, unfair? You don't get to choose how you are born into the game, but you can decide how you want to play. It's more constructive that way.

So, what *DID* you sign up for?

How many of us have heard or said, "I didn't sign up for this!" It's effortless to point out the things we don't want:

We do not want to lose.

We do not want to be the last pick.

We do not want to be unhappy.

We don't want to fail.

We don't want to be lonely.

We don't want to be broke... or broken.

Your aversion to pain ironically has you seeking it out or experiencing more of it. Again, the irony thing all up in our faces!

If you can think back to your earliest memory about your grown-up future, what and who did you want to be? How did that future image of yourself change as you got older? Did you want to be an entrepreneur or work for a big company? Was performing more your jam? Possibly an athlete or entertainer? Some of you may have had a more traditional image: marriage, children, and a home in which to grow old. All of those are great expectations. (Hmm, that's an excellent title for a book!) What compromises did you make along the way? Did you compromise to achieve a dream or lower your expectations? (If you are under the age of 21, ask your parents the previous questions. If you are older than 21–ask your parents the previous questions!).

Our future-telling is incomplete at best. Many of our expectations are overwhelmingly focused and dependent on external and often out-of-control outcomes. We then double down on this habit and base our subjective well-being on our outcomes. Have you ever caught yourself saying, "I'll be happy when...?" It's like when they say in sports, "You're only as good as your last game." Damn! Really? You suck when you lose, and you're fantastic when you win, huh? That's a dubious recipe for success, and it'll wreak havoc on your motivation. It's also a very dumb and dangerous habit for play-ing the game of life, because none of us are immune to losing, even when you are the best.

Delayed gratification doesn't mean you have to suffer in the meantime. You are allowed to enjoy getting there, even though there may be some suffering along the way. You can be happy even though you struggle to attain whatever you are working to earn. The pursuit of happiness is not the pursuit of a feeling but rather a quest to live up to an ideal. Hopefully, it's one that you have created, and as you move toward that ideal and get closer to it, you will be happi-er. What might be missed — or harder to grab a hold of — is that there is (or can be) happiness in the pursuit itself. The ugly rub is, there is no guarantee you'll meet your goal or get the gold at that end of the rainbow. Our natural wiring tells us to feel sorry for ourselves when we're getting our asses kicked. We are all susceptible to the seduc-tion of the pity party. Feeling sorry for ourselves tends to keep us in loss mode *and* have us feeling significant at the same time. It is easy to let our problems define us. Victimhood is big these days. There are lots of people selling it and buying it. I promise you, buying or selling it will not work well for you in the long run, even if you have in all reality been victimized. Regardless of your life stage, accepting and taking on the challenge to live up to your dreams will only make you more formidable. That in and of itself is a win. And one can, at the very least, appreciate that. Gratitude may not be happiness, but it's a damn close second.

None of us chose to be born. We did not sign up for life. Yet, we cannot deny the fact that we are here. As with any game, there's a set of rules that regulate how you conduct yourself while playing the game. Since you're here anyway, why not play this thing well? As with any game, there are things you'll want to know and things you'll want to do in order to put some points on the board.

Real observation:

We sometimes "need" the conflict to feel significant.

Truth is:
Your significance is not predicated on your suffering.

Essential Truths

But like rules, it's up to you to accept and follow them.

You don't have to. You better want to!

You do have choices. It may seem that you "have to" do something, but it's ultimately up to you to accept the task in front of you. It's all elective. The prisoner of war does not have to give up the secret location. It just seems like they made her do it. There was, after all, a gun pointed at her head. It may feel like someone else is making you do something, but what is making you do a thing — anything — is your own ambition, guilt, obligation, sense of responsibilities, and more.

As a kid, I had many excuses for why I didn't take out the trash, or why something might have been unfair or unjust. As an athlete, I came up with a multitude of reasons why I shouldn't have to train in certain ways. As a student, there were plenty of great reasons to explain the absurdity of taking a foreign language that was based in grammar versus conversation. No good reasons to "have to" do those things. However, while it was a rule that I had to take out the trash, crack off some road miles, and take three semesters in a foreign language, no one pointed a gun to my head. If I wanted to go out on the weekend, taking the trash out was a good idea. If I wanted to have some semblance of a good year of racing with enough in the tank for the end of the year, doing the base training made sense. If I wanted to graduate college, getting through the core requirements would be nice. I didn't "have to" do any of those things.

We all have the choice to do otherwise. Sure, some choices are easier or harder to make than others. No, you don't have to go to work for the rest of the week, but how would that turn out for you if you didn't go? You also don't have to work out, read to your young children, or keep up with your favorite hobbies, but how does that turn out for you? You don't have a gun pointed to your head. Many of us act as if we are under the gun, and have no choice. But you do have the freedom to choose within certain frameworks and contexts. Exercise the fact that you do choose, everyday. If you are not happy with your set of choices, the framework, or the context, then let's get to work on choosing a different set-up. Hard? Yes. Guaranteed? No. If you want to change the set-up, just remember: you don't have to, but you better want to.

The struggle, in many cases, is manufactured.

There is a term we use in psychology called secondary gain. Secondary gain is "the advantage that occurs to a stated or real illness." (Davidhizar R. The pursuit of illness for secondary gain. Health Care Superv. 1994 Sep;13(1):10-5. PMID: 10172109.) The reasons for secondary gains are psychologically complex. However, in *very* general terms, they stem from unmet needs. In the case of manufacturing struggle, at least outside of the legitimate medical/psychological diagnostic sense, many of us still tend to benefit from our struggle. There is a slight feeling of importance from "trying everything" and having none of it work. The very thing that ails us starts to give us meaning and identity. If we lose that thing to complain about, what excuse will we have? What will be the foundation for the future failures we will endure? It has to be existential or systemic, because our egos or insecurities cannot bear to face our shortcomings.

People get hurt. You can get sick. In most crimes, there is, in fact, a victim. Pain is real. But our struggles, in many cases, come from the avoidance of pain rather than from the pain itself. Remember, our problems can become our platforms.

If your job is getting in the way of your work, then you may have a problem.

Most would think that one's job is the same as one's work or vice versa. Your "work" is a body or group of actions that serve a bigger purpose or aim. For instance, Steve Jobs' work was about changing how the world uses technology and simplifying technology for the masses. The "jobs" for Jobs (bad dad joke intended) were the to-do's along the way to achieve his higher aims. If your jobs—i.e. the tasks on your to-do list—do not contribute to the more significant purpose, then there is a problem. Don't let it become your platform!

It's up to you to reconcile if what you are doing daily, weekly, monthly, or yearly contributes to the legacy you want to leave behind. There are things we do for money. Some of us trade time for money, while others trade value (expertise, knowledge, skills) for payment. Your work is also inclusive of what you do outside of your profession. The types of relationships you've created and how people feel when they are around you are part of your work. The habits or routines you employ, the family traditions you observe, and how you share these things are also part of your work. Lastly, as it relates to what you like to do outside of your career and family—your passions, hobbies, interests, etc.—those are part of your work, too. Bear in mind, your hobbies and interests may not pay, but it is in your best interest to design a life where whatever you are exchanging for money can pay for your passion. Jobs are what you do. Your work is what you are are building.

There is one thing getting in the way of what you say you want. Here are two questions for you:

    1. What is it you fear?

    2. What lies are you telling yourself? (Hint: They usually show up in the form of excuses.)

The answers to both of those questions will reveal what's getting in the way of what you want. Scientific limitations do exist.

You're not going to jump off a building and magically fly. We do live in societies with laws. However, we can argue that illegality only makes a behavior unsavory in the law's eyes, rather than not possible. Outside of things we cannot control, the one thing in your way are your beliefs. Your beliefs about the world. Your beliefs about others. Your beliefs about you.

What are your beliefs? How did they get there? Did you consciously decide, "This is what I believe?" Or are some of those beliefs convenient explanations for things unknown or too complicated to get into right now? The last question isn't a question. None of them were, except the first. All of it is really a question of importance or priorities.

As it pertains to what you say you want, it could be a competition of priorities. Your beliefs are rooted in many things — culture, environment, luck of the draw, personal choice, etc. You know this. What happens when your beliefs don't support or match up with what you want in the context of your priorities? For instance, your belief regarding success (or successful people) may not match with your actual ability to succeed. Survivors' guilt applies to more than just the person who made it out of the plane wreckage. It can apply to those on the precipice of making it out of a ghetto or an unhealthy relationship. It could very well be that it's more important to be accepted by your peers than to be the first to go to college. Intellectually, a person may know that's not the case, but from a priority-belief-behavioral standpoint, it's the reason they say, "You can take the boy out of the ghetto, but you can't take the ghetto out of the boy." Feel free to insert any gender in reference to the person, and any place, situation, or circumstance for the word ghetto. People are complex, but all of us go through most of the same sh*t. <—That's a bonus essential truth for you!

The bottom line: if you don't believe you have the time, there will never be enough time. If you don't think you belong, you will most likely not get along. If you believe people don't get it, or accept it, you will find a way for them not to get it or accept it. Ironically, you get to be right all of the time. Alas, being right may not always guarantee you a win, or your freedom, or your own well-being. Ask any successfully and happily married couple.

You are unique, but your BS is nothing new

That one thing that gets in your way—that belief—is BS, and nothing new. We have all been guilty of allowing our BS to get in the way of our progress.

Admit it, at one time or another, you have thought:

I can't.

That's not possible.

There's no time.

You need money to make money.

I'm not good enough.

I don't deserve _____. (*Different than earned!)

Too old.

Too young.

Every person on the planet has unique strengths and personality traits. This, coupled with inherent talents, perspectives, experiences, values, upbringing, and interests, and we can see diversity extends beyond skin color, sexual orientation, or gender identity. Each person represents much more than what another person can see.

Excuses are limitless in quantity but limited in quality. The same goes for the belief system that doesn't allow you to move forward more healthily and happily. Remember, you get to be right all of the time. You might want to make sure you are right about how you can do something vs. the reasons why you can't.

It's hard to pay now. It hurts to pay later. Either way, you pay!

Indentured servitude is a big business. Slavery may be illegal in the United States, but I would argue many of us end up serving a master in some way, shape, or form. The question is, for what and to whom is it worth being in debt?

The concept of compounding interest is powerful and translates beyond financial investments. I've had countless conversations with young professionals and pre-professionals about the benefits of taking a percentage of any earned income and placing those funds in an interest-bearing account. It's a way of practicing discipline and delayed gratification. It is also a great way to ensure long-term financial success. However, the push-back from many is that they don't think they have enough to invest. In other words, it is hard for that person to pay now. However, once retirement age hits, and you don't have the funds to support yourself, how much will that hurt?

Many of you live life on credit. It's actually needed to make the big purchases in life. Some of you may abuse it to pay for things you do not need. Apart from the car, house, and frivolous purchases, the modern human can go into debt on their health and wellbeing, too. We forgo playing the game to sit at home and watch the game. We tell ourselves we will work on our side hustles next week or when we have "free time." Ironically, living on credit means you are taking some form of value now with the expectation that you will pay later.

It hurts to go back to the gym after not having gone for over a decade. It hurts to apologize to your adult children for not being a better parent. It hurts to tell your kids *they* have to go into debt if they want to finish school. Opportunity cost is inevitable. Do your best to scrap the things that will not add to your life and invest in the things that bring returns. You can pick what gets thrown out of the plane before you take off. Otherwise, when the proverbial excrement hits the fan, you may find some of the things you didn't realize you valued have already been jettisoned. Are you going to jump out of the plane to go after them? Don't answer that if you're a certified skydiver!

Your time has always been NOW.

According to definition, patience is the capacity to accept or tolerate delay, trouble, or suffering without getting angry or upset. After countless interviews and conversations with people, I can anecdotally report with a great deal of confidence that patience is hard for those who consistently make efforts to an end and much harder for those who are not making those efforts.

Whether you are working toward a life goal or find yourself lacking your true north, it will feel like your timing is off if things are not going your way. I'm not going to say there aren't magical moments when the planets align, and a person can seemingly do no wrong, but I will say you can leave room for that magic moment—just don't bet on it!

If you were to bet on someone, would it be the one working consistently toward his goal, or the other guy not making any efforts? At this point, you might even say, "Yep, the one working hard, his time will come." You might even go further to say about the aimless guy, "His time will never come." And no one would argue either of your points. The simple math for both the hard worker and the lost boy is that their time(s) have always been now. We all have the same time in the day/week/month/year, and none of us know how much time we have left. We can imagine those magical moments because we have seen so many—your favorite athlete making the play before the buzzer, or the cinderella story of the entrepreneur/influencer you follow who sold for billions or went IPO. It all certainly seemed like it was their time.

Time is an important resource for all of us, but none of us

know how much time we've been given. This is why no one can truly pay you enough for YOUR time. We use time as a unit of measure for money, when in actuality you get paid for the value provided within that time. You do something that many cannot do or won't do, and you get paid more. You do something that anyone can do, and you get paid less. Either way, It. Is. Your. Time. The proof is in the math. From birth until you return to earth, that is your time. Your time is now, because you are here now.

Pay to play. Play to win. Paid to play.

There is a difference between getting paid and making money. It's akin to the difference between rich and wealthy. Regardless of your chosen game, it will take investment on your part if you want to play for real. Time, money, energy, and in some cases, other people's resources, are necessary. There is no getting around the fact that there is always a cost associated with your elected endeavors. You would also be correct if you reasoned there are costs related to activities you wouldn't elect to do. Those costs will always exist, because there is something else you could be doing when engaged in whatever it is you chose, or feel forced, to do. Education and training cost money and time. The guitar, the drone, the mountain bike, and the art supplies all have costs associated with them. Relationships require an investment of time, attention, and yes, money, too — predicated, of course, on your dating habits or expectations of yourself as a provider. While we commit our resources to one thing, we ultimately forego the opportunity to apply those same resources to another. Opportunity requires payment, regardless of when or how.

Many of us get into something because it's fun, or we're "good at it." Some choose our career paths based on legacy, "It's just what us Richardsons do." In other cases, we find ourselves doing what is convenient (using that term loosely!) — taking an opportunity because it happened to present itself, or it was all we knew at the time. No judgment on my part, here... I mean, how can we know what we don't know? There are plenty of well-adjusted people who built great lives for themselves taking these routes. I suspect many of those well-adjusted people employed a happenstance/legacy/convenience model, albeit implicitly rather than explicitly.

Now that you see the costs, it's the playing to win part that can get a bit dicey. After conducting countless interviews, conversations, and clinical encounters, a common thread I see emerge regarding a person's dissatisfaction with life, or themselves, is stagnation. It may not be the common thread, but a common thread. That stagnation stems from a lack of clarity, lack of purpose, or both. It also stems from exhaustion. It's not that we stagnate because of depression, anxiety, or no motivation, though those can be causes. We stop moving because we did not plan any further than our point of stagnation. In other words, as you were "doing what you were good at," doing what "us insert-your-last-name-here do," and paying your bills based on the previous opportunities presented, something happened along the way. You won the game or got good enough to keep that game going. But, that game was limited.

Finding any amount of success or achievement does incredible things for you and your brain. Once you see that things seem to be working, especially toward a worthwhile end, you become more encouraged to press on. Then one day — it's not really *one* day, but one day — you get there. And once there, it might feel good to sit within the known entity of the game you just won. You're doing your thing, you're getting paid, you're able to take care of responsibilities... possibly even other people. You made it — paid to play. The thing you set out to do is happening and working at the same time. You've even developed a level of mastery in the process of your endeavors.

But that one day becomes several months, or years. Decades even. As we are taking care of our business, meeting our obligations, we get to a point where we're stuck, while others are moving forward. Meanwhile, we're trapped reacting to what is coming at us daily. At least, that's the perception and (your) subjective reality. Objectively, what just happened didn't just happen It took months and years to develop into a rut. Ruts, or "stuckness," can happen at any income level and are not confined to race, privilege, or lack thereof. Playing to win gets dicey because we sometimes set our finish lines too soon, and once we cross them, we eventually realize we are looking (and needing) another one for which to shoot. You don't articulate it as such, but it shows up in your mood, your health, and your results — eventually. Playing to win is achieving what you have defined as wins within whatever endeavor you are involved in, and then getting in the habit of setting your finish lines further out. Playing to win is about playing in a way that keeps allowing you to play.

You can win a chess match on a micro level, but your life is full of chess matches. Learning the pieces, which direction they move, and the rules are only the beginning. Chess masters understand both the simplicity and complexity of the game. They are also well aware of how their opponents play. When you reach a certain level, there are payoffs. That is getting paid to play. However, if we do not reinvest back into the game or another game, the cycle ends, and we level out. More importantly, as you approach mastery at any given thing, you will undoubtedly come across opportunities within and just outside of the mastered domain. Recognize this is an inflection point. It's an invitation to play in a larger sandbox. Despite the invite, it will still cost to play. Despite the game, you will want to identify what a win looks like for you. Once you begin to see some wins, you will recoup your investment.

Before we move on, there is one last point on this subject. There is an infinite number of games you can play in this much larger game of your life. Please recognize, by no means am I trying to make light of your existence on earth by using the words "play" and "game." The point is you are here, and by default, you are in it (the game). If you're keen on the patterns and understand them as fundamental or archetypal, you can conduct yourself (play) accordingly. Your life IS much more than a game, and that's THE VERY REASON you want to play it as best as you can!

Somewhere, someone else with a lot less than you is doing a lot more than you.

As a general rule, it's good practice not to count other people's money. In today's political climate and social media landscape, it's easy to see what others have and what you don't. More specifically, what others get and what you give. Or, what others take and what you sacrificed. You choose which of the last three sentences resonate with you the most. It's also hard not to compare yourself to the competition, neighbor, influencer, or leader in any chosen domain.

When you go out to eat, you don't order everything on the menu. You pick what you like or what sounds appetizing. Sometimes, you'll even ask to hold the onions and add extra cheese. The point here is that we choose to use what is available to us, and in some instances, we choose not to use what is available. In the case of someone with meager beginnings, it is a matter of being resourceful despite one's minimal resources. We often think we cannot achieve our goals because we lack *all* the ingredients. What many don't realize is nobody has or starts with ALL the ingredients. The other reality is, your favorite restaurant doesn't have everything on the menu. Your favorite grocery doesn't have everything in the aisles. So why do you get upset or discouraged because you lack everything (you think) you need to succeed? You learned to walk. You learned to speak, read, do math, etc. Maybe there's more to learn, earn, and do *AS* you move toward your achievements? Somewhere, someone is making a play. Whether they're in jail right now, whether they're in a basement, in rehab, or homeless—someone is making a play, right now!

It's a privilege AND a burden—or maybe—responsibility!?
Your age.

Your skin color.

Your birth order.

Your manhood.

Your womanhood.

Your identity.

Your chosen identity.

Your discovered identity.

Your inherent talents.

Your interests.

Your relationships.

Your job.

Your welfare. (all of us receive some, by the way!)

Your education.

Your citizenship.

Your immigration status.

Your political affiliation.

Your choice to change your political affiliation.

Your opinions.

Your perspectives.

Your health.

Your education.

Your street-smarts.

Your knowledge.

Your life.

Your responsibility.

Look, I know I'm threading a needle here, flirting with offending and possibly sounding like I'm unsympathetic. There is no denying some groups are better off than others financially, socially, historically. I am not here to argue the merits of democracy, the pitfalls of socialism, or champion any particular group or movement. I admonish arbitrary hate, exclusion, as well as most things that only amount to appearance, shallow rhetoric, and virtue signaling. It gets tricky, though. Words such as "arbitrary," "surface," "shallow," and "virtue-signaling" shouldn't give away my "position," but in a politically charged climate, ALL of the terms we use seem to place others in a group or on a "side."

If you're working to box me in, it's not entirely your fault. Our brains like order. We cannot stand cognitive dissonance. If something isn't matching up, you will naturally and unconsciously work to make it match up by way of placing things within a model or framework that makes sense to you. If you are consciously trying to find fault in what I am saying, you most likely will. It's not politically correct or even polite, but based on human behavior and based on human history, we are improving. The proof is not that we've run out of problems, but rather the specificity and granularity of the problems with which we contend. We went from problems of access to problems excess. It is useful to take a critical look at social ailments and any issue that affects society. However, the sky is not falling. Why? Because it can't.

There are benefits of belonging, community, and shared experience. Enjoying those benefits are a privilege. There is also a responsibility that comes with belonging—that community, and that shared experience. I happen to be part of a minority group, one that has historically been oppressed and purposely left out or sabotaged. Yet, I would have it no other way. Why? Despite our tumultuous past in this United States of America, I also recognize that it's a great privilege to be part of such a rich history. From slave-trade to the presidency. From British-India to the White House. What a privilege — and responsibility. The truth is, we all bear burdens. Unfortunately, some way more than others. Still, even though you may belong or identify as (_____), I am willing to bet you are also more than the sum of your total parts, experiences, and how you identify. We can be "part of," and "more than," at the same time.

Not everyone will like seeing you win. Some of those reasons may be well-founded, while other reasons stem from:

Ignorance — they just don't know, and it's not always their fault.

Fear — somehow many believe that you doing well means they will not. And...

Resentment — they are not where you are, yet wish they were.

While ignorance, fear, and resentment are natural occurrences in our feelings spectrum, falling prey to them — letting them guide you rather than inform you — only stunts your ability and efficacy if not properly dealt with.

"Properly dealing" with these things is seeking a therapist, mentor, or qualified coach to help you understand your behavior, actions, and results. *If you find that your mood or general disposition makes it hard for you to function on a daily or weekly basis, please seek trained medical or clinical help.*

You are not scared of failure.

The real fear is having your negative beliefs validated.

Here's the trick: accept you can fail and work to change your belief.

This is the fight.

J

#morebetterhappier

5

4 Reasons You Might not be Getting What You Want

Sometimes it gets worse before it gets better.

Reason #1 - You just might not be doing enough.

You are not working the third shift. The third shift is that time you have after you finish your day job (or school day). It's when most of your world is asleep in bed, and you have time to yourself. It could be the wee hours in the morning or late at night. That is the third shift. That off-time can be used to put something into play.

This is not a "rise and grind" comment, and I'm not looking to guilt you into turning off the TV or bringing your laptop on vacation. This IS to say, however, that you probably have time — dare I say chunks of time — that can be used to work toward your higher aims. If you can pragmatically take the extra 5, 10, 25, or 45 minutes to "work on" whatever you want to work on, that time will amount to something.

Reason #2 - You stopped short.

You might already be doing "the extra." You might be doing everything you can — working a third shift, and even a fourth — but, reason two is about pulling out too soon. You literally quit digging just before you struck oil, or gold, or whatever the big payoff is for you. Look, I know you have obligations. Many of those obligations are about taking care of others. Why would anyone sacrifice or risk what they have going now to pursue something that's not guaranteed? All of those are legitimate reasons to pull back, reassess, or quit on your dream. I don't say that in a guilt-you-into-doing-more-stuff-way. I respect conscious decisions. There will be a time for all of us to put down the sword.

Ultimately, you never *really* know. It could be just around the corner. There are far more with far less doing a lot more than you. This isn't about selling all your possessions or quitting your job to pursue a dream. This is about making sure you keep working toward your dream. Part of working toward those dreams is continuing to refine them as you chip away in large OR small chunks. Lastly, many of you look at what you would be giving up to continue. Valid point. I am asking, what do you give up when you give up?

Reason #3 - You just really don't want what you say you want.

Have you ever found yourself saying, "It'd be nice to have...?"

"It'd be nice to win the lottery!" But you don't buy a ticket (nor should you make a habit of it!).

"It'd be nice to go on that vacation some day!" But you haven't set a date.

"It'd be nice to lose more weight, gain more muscle, make more money..." But, eating habits, exercise habits, and work habits are still the same.

It could be that your dreams are not really yours. Plenty of you are living a life — or planning a life — that someone else wants for you. Plenty of you are setting goals based on a normative standard of success. That is, you're aiming for "where you should be" based on everyone else's idea of success. And while a certain house, car, job, neighborhood, waist size, etc., might be nice, are those things what *you* want?!?! Check in with yourself. Do you really want what you say you want? Otherwise, it's just talking or living a life that is not yours. Paying attention to what is lacking as you verbalize some ideal that you're not working toward is the equivalent to expecting to hit a ball better with no batting practice.

I get it. We all have connections with others, and none of us want to let our people down. Endeavoring to do that is noble for sure. But who said there weren't costs associated with our goals? Who's life are you living? Is this the life you want? Again, you can move as fast or slow as you please, be disruptive to your status quo, or make incremental progress. My hope is you are working toward some sense of your own ideal life. While many may think you should use your education to get a great job on Wall Street, you might be happier using what you have learned and applying it in a rural community. While you might even think you would like to sit on the beach and drink fruity alcoholic beverages, you might find paying for adventure-cations more suited to you and what you value.

If you are working hard to check boxes that are not your own (beyond the honey-do list), you may find time moving faster than you like. You may find yourself becoming resentful. Ironically, those you are trying to appease may not find much quality in their time spent with you. There is room to do what's right *and* what's right for you. Not everyone will like it, but they will definitely respect it. Figuring out what you want is key. It will be easier to move in that direction once you have the vision or ideal in your mind… and heart.

Reason #4 - You're not good enough.

Yes, I said it… But, keep reading!

Maybe you are sticking with it. Maybe you're working toward the things you want. You might even be going above and beyond as it pertains to effort and time. So please don't take this the wrong way. But, it could be that you're *not* good enough. I don't mean not good enough as a person or not capable—just not good enough… yet!

There are levels to these things:

When I was a kid racing BMX, all I wanted was to be a factory-sponsored rider, which meant traveling the US racing for points in a national series, representing some big bicycle brand. When I started racing, I was not very good. It took me three years to move into the expert category (factory riders are experts and pros, BTW). After I turned expert, it took several years to be competitive locally, then state-wide, and about six years into my expert career, nationally. Then one day...

I'll never forget it! I won a national event in Ventura, Calif., and Harry Leary (google "Harry Leary BMX") came over to talk to me. He offered me a free Diamond Back bike with the possibility of being on the team. The next few months consisted of me making many national event finals on that bike. All the while, I'm thinking it's finally going to happen. I'm gonna ride for the legendary Diamond Back team! Until

It didn't happen. Despite my effort, they decided to put another kid on the team. There were several factors involved in the decision, but the main factor was this: The kid they chose instead of me didn't just make all of his main events, he was winning them. The truth was, I didn't perform well enough to merit a spot on that team. They weren't looking for a kid that could win. They were looking for a kid on that team that was winning. I wasn't good enough, as evidenced by the fact that I wasn't putting it together consistently enough for the level I wanted to play.
Until

I started winning more consistently. The way to winning more consistently was doing more and becoming better—riding, practicing, and working on my race craft. By winning more consistently, I eventually proved to be good enough to merit the big sponsorship. Was it with my buddy Harry and the Diamond Back team? No. It with another brand—and several other notable brands thereafter.

Like I said, there are levels to this. Anyone can get lucky once or twice. However, over time, the luckiest tend to be the most dedicated, ready, and prepared.

You don't need anyone's approval...

But...you will generally get it once you approve of yourself.

True story

J

6

Essential Questions

*Who knew 8th grade Language Arts
serves to guide our lives?*

Do you want to protect your ego, or do you want to be happy?

Be mindful that prideful doesn't necessarily lead to "proud."
Unfortunately, all of us can fall between even the finest of lines. Exhibiting pridefulness leads us not to ask for help when we need it and tricks us into thinking we know what the other person is talking about before they finish their sentence. Pridefulness may also lead us down a path that is not our own. And that's the rub — it *is* your path, whether you

are being led by your ego, your logic, your heart, or someone else.

The curious thing about protecting your ego is you ultimately still know where you are. It's like lying about your age. You know how old you are! Most of you anyway. There are some who don't due to the lack of record keeping back in the day. Regardless of how young you look, it's kinda sad to see the old dude in the club. Ultimately, that's trivial. Have you ever avoided feedback? The A, B, or C-list celebrity who needs their entourage? Too proud to ask for help? Need to be right? It's no coincidence the size of the ego is related to the size of insecurity. Seeking, or always needing, external validation sometimes has our egos making purchases we can't afford. Ego may have you keeping up with the Joneses, but it might not be in alignment with what's in your heart. And, what I mean by heart is what you know brings you more joy or fulfillment. A new car every three years is nice, but if you truly like taking the bus and Lyfting when you need it — that might be the better path for you. It's possible to be proud of what you have to offer and work toward things that improve your life (including those around you), and let that validate your self-worth or value. This is not to say you need not care what others think. This is to say that your behavior is better guided by what challenges you, gives you fulfillment, and helps you and those around you. I'm not sure that'll have you keeping up with the Joneses or Kardashians, but it will help you stay grounded as you move forward.

Will it be worth how you'll feel ON THE WAY toward (getting/having/being) what you want?

Sometimes we aren't "feeling' it," and there will definitely be times when the better decision is not to get in the ring, on the field, or track. However, if you decide to get in the ring, go on the field, or race on the track, I strongly suggest you not rely solely on how you feel. (There is, of course, way more to this, which is why working with a coach, or therapist, or mentor is so helpful. Some of those "ors" can be "ANDs" as well!)

The way you feel is *your* subjective experience and based on a multitude of external and internal factors—some explainable and some not. When you set out to do a thing, especially something that is important to you, the journey is riddled with obstacles and setbacks. You will feel discouraged at times. You will feel unmotivated, tired, frustrated, or possibly already beaten. Is it worth it? I ask you to ask yourself this question, because many of us take on things we already don't want to do—not so much in terms of responsibilities and obligations, but rather in taking on a major career or study direction. The point here is that there will be some pain associated with any pursuit, so why pursue something that is already disengaging to you? If some pain is associated with moving toward a goal, why endure the pain for something that you only moderately want, or for what's expected by others, versus the things that light you up?

Important caveat here: I recognize some of you may not have a thing that lights you up. Or, there are several things that light you up. I also recognize that what lights you up may not pay the bills. I suggest if your passion does not pay, do something that pays for your passion. From a professional standpoint, it behooves you to learn your strengths and personality traits so you can set yourself up for success. If you can play to your strengths and understand your unique personality make-up, it will help you filter out what's worth your time and/or how to approach your list (macro or micro) of to-dos'.

My wife reminds me of how miserable I was during the years I raced BMX for a living. I look back on those days with nostalgia and romance. However, she's right! My peers and I spent a great portion of those years obsessing, stressing, and worrying about our gate starts, sponsorship opportunities, the bleak payouts at some events, and what the hell we were going to do next after the racing-a-bike-thing is done. Yet, most of us loved it—and still do! The things I was working toward at the time was worth the feelings I dealt with along the way. My hope is that if you're feeling discouraged, frustrated, or just plain tired much of the time, those feelings come from the pains and obstacles associated with pursuing something of value to you—the things that light you up!

"What will I really think of myself if I don't go for it?"

It's one thing to be 18 and push something off until you are 21. It's another thing to be 30, then 40, and then 58 pushing something off, because in those middle-age years through retirement, THAT is when you will want to (and possibly need to) collect on what you "put in" when you were younger. Compounding interests plays a role here.

What I'm getting at is: What is the highest level of life that you can think possible? All of it! Your money. Your fitness. Your family. Your experiences, friends—everything. I am talking about going for that!

You may look at your life now and think, "It's not that bad," or "This is great!" I would also bet if you throw the stone out another 5, 10, 15 years, there is at least an idea, however faint it may be, of what you want your life to be. The truth is there is a part of all of us that settles and compromises. We live in a world full of people, and life can hit hard. At the very least, I want you to think about your non-starters. The stuff that is a resounding, "Hell no!" From there, be honest about where you are and what you want. What YOU want. Not just the material stuff, but the real stuff — health, people, experiences, and yes, money, too! Your best life. If you are already living that, great! Pass your secrets along to your friends and family. Lord knows, maintaining that best life will be work, too. If your best life is not what you are living, or heading toward, then this is the time to look in the mirror.

As someone connected to other people — parents, partners, siblings, family, friends, co-workers — being a person who says something and then sets out to do it is a powerful way to lead your life. For you, and for them! The irony is that despite your chosen game — or your wish to just put your head down and do your job — you'll still manage to influence others. Charles Barkley's 1993 commercial may have said he wasn't a role model, but it's definitely not 1993 anymore. We know people are (always) watching. It's nice to be liked, but that doesn't guarantee respect. If you move through life knowing you sold yourself short—and deep down you *would* know—you will have created a new premise (belief possibly?) from which you operate. That new premise may have an adverse affect on how you show up for the things that matter to you in the future. We will get into the whole "new premise" thing in the next essential question.

Lastly on this question, there is no guarantee for success. Going for it might be high risk. I want you to be responsible—I really do. Responsibility keeps you grounded and helps you become a stronger person. Be mindful, even a "safe" job can be dangerous. If you are going to spend energy, time, money to pursue a thing, it's also your responsibility to give yourself the best chance at what you think can be your ultimate life.

How do your beliefs about yourself, others, and the world, hold you back?

This is not a question many ponder. In fact, I'd wager you believe your beliefs help you cope or drive you forward. For the most part, your beliefs do get you through. As alluded to in a not so illusory manner in the *Domestic Silence* chapter, it's the (conflicting) beliefs that cause many of us to become so animated. Countries go to war because of different beliefs. Groups protest based on their beliefs. People go for the jugular on Twitter and Facebook because of their beliefs. You and and I can do extraordinary things based on our beliefs. You and I can also really screw things up based on our beliefs.

It's here that I want you to pause...

As it pertains to yourself, others, and the world, think:

"I am..."

"They are..."

"This is" or, "That is..."

Self. Others. World.

The premise (belief) from which you operate generally dictates how you will feel, what you'll do (or not do), and what you get. The chain of events is as follows:

B e l i e f s — > F e e l i n g s — > A c t i o n s — > R e s u l t s
Self

If I'm in sales and believe, "I am not capable of meeting my goals," how does that play out for me? Feeling nervous, stressed, possibly unmotivated? Slow to get on calls or, perhaps, calling too much? How often am I checking in with my team to stay accountable? Based on my beliefs, feelings, and actions related to meeting my sales goals, what would you say are my results? As Ricky Gervais would say, "F**k all!"

Others

Perhaps you have a strong sense of self, and you believe you *can* get the job done. But, you are part of a team, and your belief about your peers is, "They don't work as hard as they should (or me!)." If you believe your team doesn't work as hard as they should, you might feel resentful, angry, and frustrated. Those feelings may lead you to lash out at your teammates or possibly even throw them under the bus to clients or co-workers. That kind of action will earn you distrust amongst your team along with a poor team result, and YOU falling short of the goal by proxy.

World

You might believe both you and your team are solid. But we're in a global pandemic, and everyone on the team is operating on the premise that "It's impossible to get anything done—no one is selling or buying!" Who's going to feel motivated? Who's going to wake up earlier or stay up a bit later to work? What results do you expect based on this scenario? By the time you read this, you may have your answers to those questions. It is still playing out.

Meanwhile, someone out there believes they're capable of

meeting their goals. Maybe others don't work as hard as you. But they could be doing the best they can, and/or working smarter than you! And, despite a global pandemic, things can get done, albeit in different ways and on adjusted timelines. Lastly, don't confuse hope for belief. Belief drives action. Hope, while it is comforting and warranted, is more like a passenger than a driver.

"What advice do I give others that I, myself, do not follow?"

See? You're probably more brilliant than you credit yourself. Or you think your problems are too special or unique to trust that what you say will work for others might work for you!
Or... You don't believe in the poop you are scooping.

If the former is the case, then get to work on what you tell others to work on! If the latter is the case, stop giving advice and take some good advice from people you respect and challenge you. It goes without saying that the best way to receive good advice is to act on that advice. So I won't say it... even though I just did.

"What can I do to win the day?"

If you're young, it may feel like you have plenty of time. You're most likely driven by passion and heart. Doing the things you want to do. Hopefully, the things you do now are also moving you toward a life you want for yourself. If you're older (middle-age and beyond), it probably seems that time goes faster with each passing year. What might be driving you are deadlines, obligations, and making up for bad choices when you were young.

Whether old or young, today was once yesterday's future. The journey is long, and it will be over before you know it. Take the time to ask yourself what you can do to win the day today, tomorrow, and the next. At the very least, ask yourself once a week, and hit each day with a bit of intention. Give yourself a couple of pins to knock down! This will prove to be one of the best habits you can create for yourself. There could be plenty of things on your list that would allow you to "win the day," but can you narrow it down to three things? Hopefully, they have something to do with your wealth, health, and happiness—it doesn't have to be that order.

"What do I get once I get what I want?"

There are plenty of people who got what they said they wanted. The promotions. The medals. The successful business. But for some of them, it just wasn't quite what they thought. Purpose drives resiliency, meaning we can go a long way in dealing with adversity and pain if or when we are moving toward a goal. In many cases, this *is* a way to cope with your more internal psychological and emotional struggles—finding something to work toward and seeing it through can distract you from focusing on your perceived shortcomings. Therapeutically speaking, working toward a goal builds you up psychologically and emotionally. You develop useful habits. You get opportunities to solve problems, which in turn, show you that you are capable. But it's a matter of meaning. What will it mean to, or for, you? Right? There is a reason why you want what you want.

There is something called Mimetic Desire, coined by Rene Girard (1923-2015), a former professor at Stanford University. We (sometimes) don't know what we want, so we imitate the wants of others. This effect has many of us thinking we are in competition for the same things, ultimately ending in a battle of sorts (my over-simplification, not his words) or rivalry based on who's getting/having and who's not getting/having. I am adding that the battle (or rivalry) takes place within ourselves as well. It comes down to validation. At what point will you be good enough? Is it their acceptance of you, or your acceptance of you?

It's not the car we want. It's the experience or possibly the status. With experience or status comes a feeling. The former, more visceral, the latter, more ephemeral. It's not the job or money we want. It's the freedom, or perceived power. Maybe control is the better word. Generally speaking, when we look to something external, it's not that thing we want. It's what we think we will get when we get what we want.

At what point will you cross the threshold from just getting by to thriving? And when I say, "just getting by," I do mean that relatively. Our brains are looking to keep us alive. Much of our neurological programming from our early existence as a species is still working quite well. However, survival—from an ego standpoint, from a sense of self-worth standpoint, from a sense of well-being standpoint, from a relational standpoint, and career, and happiness, and on and on —- exists in many ways along the spectrum of socio-economic or power structure hierarchies. Many are looking for something. If it's not the car, the job, or even the six-pack abs, what is it? It's not just *one* thing, but many of you don't think that's the case

Your ideals will become someone else's if not acted upon.

J

P.S.
...and that someone else will deserve them!

#morebetterhappier

Congruence

"Life is a beautiful struggle

People search through the rubble for a suitable hustle

Some people usin' the noodle, some people usin' the muscle

Some people put it all together, make it fit like a puzzle"

Talib Kweli

7

One Thing

...it's never just one thing.

According to Sigmund Freud, we live the good life when we work, play, *and* love. In this instance, I agree with my preoccupied-with-mommy-and-daddy-issues predecessor. The typical cycle for many Americans, and first-world-westernized nations, is this: We are born. We go to school. Then we go to more school (to get a job). We start families (or get a dog). We send our kids to school. They get jobs. They start families. They send their kids to school. They get jobs. And so on. This is the current model. Born, school, and then, get a job, only to pass on the tradition.

Aside from the school part, picking what we want to do part, and having the ability to think about our own thoughts and behavior part, most living organisms do the same things — go through their lives with a non-conscious objective of living. Growth, movement, reproduction, respiration, nutrition, and excretion. We humans, get the added bonus of choosing how we want to do this. One could argue that the thinking part of us, the "meta" part, is part of the design as well. I would argue that point... but I am neither an evolutionary biologist, nor is this "letter" written to debate why we think or have the ability to be aware of ourselves in a way that seems beyond most other living organisms. I point this out to say that as part of a living breathing planet, we too, are governed by certain universalities just like the rest of nature. So, if we are hardwired to keep living (as individuals and species), but we also have this awareness allowing us to rate the quality of our existence (whether by design or not), how best can we maximize the totality of it all? What does that even look like?

Right around high school age is when I remember all of those, "You need to buckle down" conversations. I too, am guilty of that same conversation with my kids, albeit nuanced and more to the point of asking them to think about the kind of life they want for themselves (sorry guys... kinda). The truth is, at some point, everyone is going to want to figure out how to get by on their own. Based on my observation and thousands of interviews, I've noticed if you don't figure out a way to get by, it will be figured out for you. I am using "getting by"—again—in the most relative of terms, and as a baseline at the same time.

In my conversations with clients and others in a helping or service profession, I, along with my colleagues, have noticed that most people seem to want everything to be fixed, yet fixate on one thing. Usually, the one thing is career/work. That makes sense, since our work should provide for the necessities of food, clothing, and shelter. Our work also provides/dictates a lifestyle. Whether that lifestyle is by default or demand is where More. Better. Happier. plays the proverbial field and where we are going next.

Most people assume there is only so much room at the top. Most people accept sayings like, "You can't win every time." One trope movie makers and news media like to perpetuate is that of the noble underdog. Most people think... like most people. And, most people aren't thinking about the whole field. Most people can't win every time, but they can win more times than they think. Especially if they take the time to define their wins.

Love him or hate him, what if Tom Brady thought like most

people?

Flat-Earther or not, what if Einstein thought like most people?

Beliefs about vaccinations and billionaires not paying their fair share aside, what if Gates, Branson, and Winfrey thought like most people?

Many of us see *those people* as special, or lucky, and they are lucky, actually. You may see those people as being bigger than life, or possessing extraordinary talent, and that might be true, as well. I've touched, ahem—HARPED—on this before in my talks and previous writings, but those people are just like you. I promise you. They once started out as kids from Mississippi, or San Mateo, or Blackheath, or Ulm, Germany.

I'm just a kid from South Jersey. Growing up, some of my friends thought I was dreaming when I said I wanted to be on magazine covers and travel the world racing BMX. And they were right—I was dreaming! But, I saw it through all the way to a 15-year pro BMX career, a world championship at the beginning, a PanAm Games gold medal towards the end. Also by design, I went to school along the way and earned a few degrees. Did I win everything all of the time? No. Do I have a decent record at success? Sure. Do you have the ability to define, design, and go after what you would consider wins for you? Yes. A resounding YES!

We love to go to work on that one thing. We love to think that one thing will *work for us* once we get it! You may have even picked up this book because you're looking for that one thing. Make no mistake, I want you to have it! The whole reason I got in to the psych game was to help people get what they want. The reason clients work with me is to get that one thing...

"I want an Olympic medal!"

"I want to make a career change."

"I just want to be heard."

"I just want to be happy."

The things people want tend to fall into one of three categories:

More

This "more" domain consists of stuff. The house, car, bank accounts, jobs and titles, and the status associated with all that stuff. All the external stuff and the success that drives those material wins. This is the place where many of you hang your hats. Hopefully, not your identities. The client looking for more wants the promotion. They client looking for more wants to level up in some way that has a hard metric based on money and/or success. For this domain, think affluence.

Better.

Let's be clear, having great health insurance does not ensure great health! The "better" domain is all about your health, abilities, and capabilities. Your efficacy, if you will. The client looking for better wants to lose (or gain) the weight. They want to get stronger, more proficient, or look better in the mirror. Here is where we not only measure up, but we feel we can be more effective—more relevant—at least in our minds. For this domain, think influence.

Happier.

The "happier" domain is just that—where your relationships, experiences, and perspective reside. This is the domain of, "Is it all worth it?" Clients looking for happier tend to want to work on relationships. The client looking for happier might feel like something is missing. The client looking for happier may have to confront their feelings of rejection, worthiness, abandonment, and stress about an uncertain future. We can measure career and sports success with money, promotions, responsibilities, accolades, and points on the board. We can measure health success with kilos/pounds, blood sugar, cholesterol, VO2 max, and strength or endurance gains. The happier domain is harder to measure, yet you still know if you are "there" or not. Your experiences and relationships live in this domain. For this domain, think quality. Also, think habits. All of us can work on our habits despite our predispositions towards happiness.

Are you working toward what you are really seeking? We've learned to separate our work life from our home life. We try to separate our work life from our play life and play life from home life. Some of you move from the domestic silo to the work silo, and if you have time between the obligations of home and work, there's a very slim silo entitled "weekend" and "vacation" at best, or "alcohol" and "drugs" at worst. I thought a lot about that last sentence. The alcohol and drug silo can become a prison. The lines between use, abuse, and addiction get blurry faster than most of us think.

You've mostly likely heard someone say, "I'll be happy when..." How many of us have an if/then/when logic tree as it relates to all those "lives" we live in our silos?

"I'll be happy when I have less to do at work?"

"I'll be happy when I make partner. Then I'll have more time to get back in shape."

"If the system wasn't stacked against me, I would be better off."

"...And, I would have gotten away with it too, if it weren't for you meddling kids!

Compartmentalization is a good skill and a great tool. However, that tool may not be right for every job. Integration is a tool we forget to employ. Seeing as how life happens with or without you—and that life is often messy and complicated—integration as a tool and concept are well worth understanding. How can I integrate my work with my play? How can I integrate my family values with my work obligations? How do my interests outside of work inform and help my work? What can I take from work and apply to my other interests, or at home? To what extent is it possible to design a life that honors the fact that I am more than just my job, that my work (helps) supports my family, and that I'm pursuing my other interests? This chapter is titled "*One Thing*" because somehow we (myself included… I still work on this stuff, too!) have defined success as "*things.*" *You do* things for a living. I do things for a living. You are someTHING (doctor, lawyer, athlete). I am someTHING. We buy things, sell things, place value on things, and on and on. Work and the procurement of things has become the gold standard for success. And, why not? Things, and the measurement or accounting thereof, offer clear metrics. Money in the bank, range on your EV battery, toys in the garage, are all ways to show, measure, and hopefully enjoy success. The more we work, the more things we can get. The more things we can get, the more successful we appear.

There is a lot of time spent in the accumulation of things, and I would be lying if I said I didn't enjoy a new bike, or car, or giving someone a great gift. Yet, during our time accumulating things, we begin to realize—if we do not inherently know—that our things are not enough! Working and not playing sucks. Playing and not loving, well that leaves us a bit empty, too. All the while, those in our lives whom we do love are quite possibly immersed in their own school->work->kids-> cycle themselves.

Once we realize this pattern is not serving us, we then strive for the *one thing* that we think will solve our problem: balance. To achieve balance, we pick the one thing that we think is missing most. So, back to the list:

"I just want to make more money."

"I just need to make more time."

"The next house will be our last move."

"I just need to lose 20 pounds."

"I just want to be happy."

Balance is not about keeping things stable outside of you. Equal division of time and labor do not equate to being balanced. Balance is about you being more stable when things are not. The phrase, "We need more balance in our life," suggests it's just a matter of time management, scheduling, and giving things equal attention. As I just typed that, I think to myself, "Damn, that doesn't sound too bad." And it's not, on the surface. To me — and for you — the true meaning of the phrase is, "We need to _be_ more balanced in our life." Splitting hairs I know, but an important distinction. The problem is not balance, per se, but what our perception of balance can become. If that perception has something to do with controlling things beyond your control — creating habits that are somewhat unsustainable / untenable, having an-all-or-nothing mindset, or deep down believing you can't have it all — then you'll want to tighten your seatbelt and take something for an upset stomach. The problem of balance is not really a problem. It is a lifelong project. The project is not about wanting and getting, or living in a model of if-then-else scenarios. The project is about having vs. getting. Having everything vs. getting everything. More integration, less compartmentalization.

Yes, that's right! Having everything is all about rearranging the playing field in your head and on the ground, getting out of the silos and realizing those silos exist on a larger plot of land. Your existence is more than line items and checklists, though lists are great. The trick is to play to your strengths, learn to scaffold, do your best to be honest (refer the Rules for Engagement), and recognize that your responsibilities also include taking care of yourself, your business, AND others — not necessarily in that order. It is a blend of being and doing. If you think this is BS (bullsh*t) then maybe you're thinking in terms of stuff and line items. If you just leaned forward in your chair or pressed the little "15 sec back button" on your mobile device, then you are ready for some real BS — ⟩ Belief System. Let's go!

Okay… it really is just ONE THING

We all want more. Our brains are hardwired for more. From the Renaissance to the Industrial Revolution, to the Tech Revolution bubble, now the Digital, and going into the A.I. age (leaped there!), humans' neurological programming keeps us wanting and searching for more, and pushing boundaries. I categorized "More" as affluence, "Better" as an influence, and "Happier" as quality, based on the conversations I've had over time with people across all incomes, races, genders, etc. All pointed to these areas in their respective lives. If I am smelling my own cooking, these too have been the three areas I've tried to solve for in my own life.

But there is More, and that More is not just about stuff or things. You know this. There is Better, and it's certainly not because you obtained more of that stuff, although you might have had to become better to obtain it. You know this, too! And happier. I left this one alone on purpose just a few paragraphs ago, as I wasn't sure what your brain might do with t the word, "happier." That is, it's easy to interpret, "happy," even though I am using, "happier," with an emphasis on the "er." It's the "er" in happier that is my main concern, because I want us all to be (just a bit) happier. I have no way of knowing everyone's baseline. Due to the realities of life, and the fact that in any given population there are going to be a subset of that population with a predisposition for illness (of any type), a subset of the population living below the poverty line, and a subset of the population that experiences both. Happier, in my estimation, is more tenable than happy, though I won't rule the latter out! But still, there is happier. It seems like a small aim, but I assure you, skyscrapers are not built from top to bottom. First, you set a foundation. It's easier to build once you have a foundation.

So, while I oversimplified the categories for a clearer understanding of the framework, there is no doubt that these three things overlap. The silos are not independent of one another. Setting good boundaries is healthy for relationships, work, and play. However, we set those boundaries to keep us healthier, happier, and safer so we can function better in all areas of our life!

One the surface, we work to survive and/or to create a type of life. Some are better than others at compartmentalizing, but we all know our performance can deteriorate if one of the three things (More, Better, and Happier) is not going well. Trouble at home can make it hard to concentrate on the job. You lose your job, how happy are the spouse and kids going to be if you have to move to a different neighborhood or start buying the off-brand shoes? If your relationships are strained, or you have a habit of drinking / drugging too much, how will that play out at work and with your family in the long run? And, all of that is just on the surface level. When those three overlap in bad ways, that place where they converge is dark — poor health, failure, and emptiness. Granted, I just painted a bleak portrait, but as you know by now, I use extremes to illustrate a point.

Convergence

Your success happens where More and Better converge. If you think about it, at several points in your life, you increased your capacity to do more, learn more, and take on more. To do all of that, I suspect you got better at things — acquiring the skill, refining your talents, dealing with responsibility. Getting the more required you to become more. Becoming more required you to become better — and you also got better by becoming more.

Your health and well-being is where Better and Happier converge. You do have better in you. We all do. When you work toward that, you will find your limits. The better person (not better than the other person, but the better you) can find pride in those inherent talents and skills. The better person has the ability to say no when something is not right or doesn't fit. That solid foundation does not come without a price at times, but over time, the person with this type of conviction creates strong relationships and appreciates what they do have. This is happier.

Your fulfillment is where More and Happier converge. Taking on more and becoming more begins to have a different meaning when you do have a team that has your back and when you know people count on you. When the burdens and responsibilities become privileges, you have arrived. You, at this point, are doing something that matters.

Now that you really know what More, Better, and Happier are, it's on you to define, name, or articulate that sweet spot. That's where More, Better, and Happier converge. Whatever word you use to define that convergence, that's the one thing you want. It might even be your North Star. This is where "having everything" comes into play. For the most part, all of "this" is already in you. Are there discrepancies, disparities, and deficiencies person-to-person on an individual basis? Yes. Does that absolve you from taking stock of your life? Does that mean you can't become more, better, or happier (remember the "er")? I know it may be easier or harder for some than others. That kinda sucks. However, wouldn't you rather your life suck less than it does now? Or, if your life is great, wouldn't you rather it stay great or get better? Because it can begin to suck if you let it. Either way, it's on you to get to work. Most importantly, this is designed to get you to look at what you like and don't like in your life. The chips may be stacked against you. People do cheat, and the system might actually be rigged. As much as it is up to you to get to work, you will also want to change how you look at things, as well. If you find you cannot get over the injustices and inequities, you may find yourself subject to them.

By no means am I saying, "just get over it." I am asking you to get through it.

If you feel compelled to push back on this framework or argue the points of convergence that I laid out—that's fine. Hopefully, I've struck a nerve, and that means you're already applying these principals. If you're pushing back, I'll challenge you further to re-create another framework. How can you take it further? Make it more digestible, actionable, or comprehensive. If it helps you and others change the trajectory of your lives for the positive, I will adopt that framework myself! That is not a challenge, actually, but a hope. If you read my words and say, "I can do better," then I have done my work. Either way, you'll still want to read what's next. We're about to bring this home!

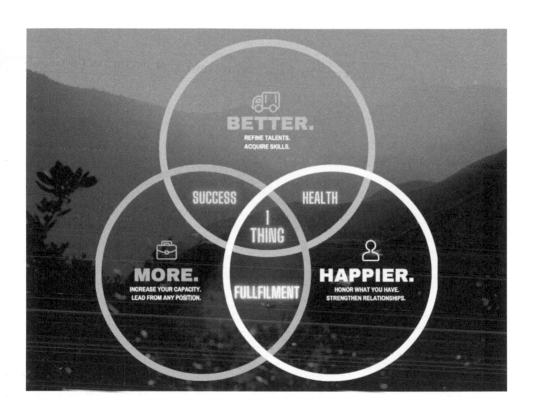

8

Play the Whole Field, Win the Whole Game

The journey is long, and it will be over before you know it!

Better not play it *too* safe, or you might be sorry.

I hate to break it to you, but you may be playing it too safe. I want to stress the emphasis on the word "too." Many of you have come a long way by NOT being reckless. Being smart and consistent accounts for compounding interest and longevity—in every facet of life. However, this is about being the dangerous one, not acting dangerously!

Do this simple exercise:

Go back to when you were maybe just out of school, begging to work in your career, or beginning a new job. What were your circumstances? What were the feelings associated with your circumstances?

My guess is you might've felt nervous, scared, stressed, doubtful—and—ready to prove yourself, willing to learn, grateful, and hopeful. There probably wasn't much to lose, but a lot to gain. That made you dangerous! Hopefully you wrote down those circumstances and feelings.

When I was competing professionally, I remember my first pro race in the same way. I was literally running scared every lap. So much so, that I found myself in contention for a top-three finish and an outside chance to win the whole thing. I ultimately ended up having a great rookie year—borne out of fear, nervousness, willingness to prove myself, and some gratitude that I made it that far.

Conversely, in the middle of my career, I had the sponsors, I had the reputation, and I also had something else—I had the fear of losing what I had. I spent the better part of three years fighting to hold on to something. It led to inconsistent performances and bouncing around trying to drum up sponsorship. Paradoxically, fighting to "hold on" to something was playing dangerously. Playing it safe cost me money, sponsorship, and almost my career. Not to mention, I wasn't as pleasant a person. Ask some of my peers. We joke about Y2k being my angry year!

The smart choice for me was to approach my training, races, and my season not with reckless abandon, but rather with a mindset of full trust. That meant I went all in **because** of what was at stake — the future I wanted, the person I wanted to be. It wasn't about the future I was trying to avoid. Promise yourself that when it's time to go all in and lay it on the line, that you actually go all in and lay it on the line. I can't guarantee you'll win each time, but I do promise this method works for winning in the long run. Of course, this is easier to do when you've tapped into some deeper meaning or passion about what you are doing.

RE:alignment

Do you like what you do? Not so much from a dream job standpoint, but more in the general scope of daily activity. Also, do you like what you do? Yes, I asked that question twice because you are more than just your job, aren't you? Or, weren't you? You know when you're watching sports and you can tell when the shot is gonna go in, the putt is good, or the ball is going out of the park? Not only are you witnessing mastery and possibly luck, you are witnessing alignment. You've heard it said many times, "The stars were aligned!" Athletes say it after a great performance, "Everything was just clicking!" When couples describe how they met, you might even hear, "The planets were aligned that night!"

I wouldn't attempt to give you some celestial explanation for success, and I can tell you that you don't have to be completely aligned to experience some success. A bit of talent and drive can take you a long way, to be fair. However, your alignment (with who you are, what type of person you want to be, and what you mean to others) has everything to to do with your total success from a framework of health, happiness, and work.

Many of us obsess about work (or school), or our hobbies, and what will make us happy or feel better in the future. Sometimes we get fixated on that one thing. Other times we are in one domain and thinking about the other. What I've noticed in people's behavior is they obsess on those things, but go to work (as in profession or job) as a fall-back or the fix. And why not? It's the easiest place to put points on the board. Much of what "you have to do" is already laid out, and our perceived chances at scoring the immediate goal seem greater.

Many of you do want it all, but don't always go for it all. Maybe because you think it's unattainable, maybe because you can't bare to try and fail, or maybe some of you have talked yourself out of how important all of it really is – *it* being addressing the better and happier portions of your existence. Now that you're thinking in terms of More, Better, Happier, think about where in your success, health, and fulfillment you want to step up your game. Better yet, give yourself a grade. How would you grade yourself in the three areas? Knowing what you know now...

Write down an answer to these three questions in each domain:

More:

What do you want to accomplish?

What do you want to do?

What type of person do you want to be?

Better:

What do you want to accomplish?

What do you want to do?

What type of person do you want to be?

Happier

What do you want to accomplish?

What do you want to do?

What kind of person do you want to be?

Just because you don't have the ball, doesn't mean the ball, or you, are not in play. Recognizing all domains are at play in your life—seeing the whole field—affords you the luxury and responsibility of more choices, better actions, and happier returns.

As an aside, many of you are closer than you think. Remember, as you move up, or on, the math works in your favor. There are fewer teams in the playoffs. There are fewer people in the second and third round of interviews. It might get harder as you get closer, but it's also simpler from an odds perspective.

Now, walk through these questions to start finding out where you might be misaligned:

First—-

Are you doing what you want to do?

If so, in what areas? If not, in what areas? And by "areas" I mean:

In your business

In your sport… or health

And, in your life (think, relationships and experiences)

Second —

What are your strengths, talents, and personality traits?

How do you utilize those strengths, talents, and traits?

How do you waste or underutilize them?

There's a lot to unpack! I suggest taking a legitimate (scientifically reliable and valid) assessment such as WorkPlace Big 5 by Paradigm Personality Labs or Clifton Strengths by Gallup to help crystalize what you might intuit about yourself. Getting guidance from a credentialed coach or therapist is also highly advised.

The purpose of this exercise is not so that you can do better on the field or in the business world. Outside of what you do for money, you still have a life. What you do for a living may occupy most of your time, but it doesn't have to define all of who you are. The artifacts that remain in your heart and mind well after having rich experiences are worth keeping, teaching, and passing down. Those artifacts include the achievements (material and otherwise) borne from the commitment to see those things through. There are far too many "successful" people feeling unfulfilled from the dollars and deals. Yet, they keep looking for wins and meaning inside of the dollars and the deals. What I would like you to ask yourself is this: *"How am I winning if I am not receiving the benefits of the win?"*

If the "touchy-feely stuff" doesn't resonate with you, fair enough. You are in it for the money. You are focused on work—as in career and getting ahead—and those things do provide meaning for you. Cool with me. Still, you should know studies have shown doodling can improve memory, exercise improves cognition, playing an instrument strengthens the part of the brain (corpus callosum) that bridges both hemispheres, and dance/sports/arts enhance executive function. So if you truly are all about business, there is plenty of proof and research to show you might be irresponsible for not tending to other areas in your life. If for no other reason than to improve your bottom line.

It is time to play the whole field again. I say again, because, at some point, many of you were probably doing just that! Remember the "Playing it too safe" bit? Some of you are lucky

enough to do what you love for a living. Many of you probably gave up things you were passionate about in order to:

Be more practical / realistic

Pay for school or rent

Focus on your career

Take the kids to their practices

Knowing what you know now — either because of what you've
read here, or because of the circumstances that led you to pick up
this book — one of the many bottom lines is this: If your passion does
not pay, it behooves you to pay for your passion. Our passions cost,
and they pay (off). The remuneration is not limited to only money. Your job pays, and it costs. Again, not limited to only money.

You may not get paid to throw a ball or dive off cliffs, but
I damn sure want you to work in a way that can afford you your
preferred lifestyle. Do you like building classic cars? Great! Do you
like competing in Spartan races? Great! Are you keen to kick it with
Elon, Jeff, or Richard, and get in some space travel? I am good with
that, too! Digging into the things you're passionate about gives you
something (More) higher for which to strive. Your day job may not
be your passion, and that's fine, but if killing it at work helps you
invest in more of your passions, then that is a win-win-win situa-

tion! If the job is killing you, how does that pay off in the long run?

You know there's something you've been putting off. You also know what you might've given up to get to where you are right now. Only you can answer if the exchanges were, are, or will be worth it. Conscious trade-offs are easier to stomach. It's the trade-offs we didn't realize we were making that bite us in the ass. Remember to check your backside for teethmarks from time to time. The ones you didn't ask for, of course!

Please keep in mind...

Some of you might be
complaining about a
current situation you
once longed for.

You don't have to make
an enemy of today to
have your tomorrow be
the hero

J

#morebetterhappier

9

Walking Strongly

How you can step up.

But, before you step up...

There are things you need to do, and things you want to do. Within that, there are things you hate doing and things you like doing. Somewhere, as you are doing (or avoiding) those things, you might find yourself spinning your wheels. This is the difference between being busy and being productive. Frankly, once you reach a certain threshold (age, income, or skill level), busy becomes a waste of your time, your team's time, and your family's time. It's the classic quantity versus quality scenario.

You may be a person with a ton of stuff to do, and ALL OF IT is important. Most of us are busy for a good reason. But, I'll push and suggest some of you might be spinning out in some areas. Here is how and why: If you're relatively responsible and relatively successful, there is a piece of you that is always working. Even if you are not "at work," your mind might be, and we know your emotions go along for the ride, as well. We are at work thinking about home. We are at home thinking about work. We are at the game thinking about home. And so on.

The way to reduce this cycle is to channel the energy you have and accept that YOU DO NOT NEED TO WORRY ABOUT THE STUFF YOU ARE GOING TO WORRY ABOUT ANYWAY! Sorry, I don't mean to yell at you. In other words, it's difficult to shut off caring about your obligations and responsibilities. This is a mindset shift. You want to trust that when you step, you are moving, even if you're not seeing movement. Stepping up is about taking what you want and reverse engineering into smaller actions and thoughts that you can control. Below is a supplementary exercise that'll help you decide — macro or micro — on what to attack, when, and possibly how: Separate your tasks into four categories:

Perform - Do this!

Postpone - Don't do this yet/now!

Assign - Get someone else to do it!

Eliminate - No need (for you) to do it!

Then, estimate:

Overestimate the time it takes to do a thing.

Underestimate how much you can get done.

Create the Most Important list (3 things) -

Anything beyond is a bonus!

Will this help eliminate late nights? Yes, but not all of them. Will this eliminate all the fires that need extinguishing? No, but some of them. Will this keep the fan spinning cleanly? Well, I would say cleaner, with emphasis on the "er." Do the little exercise above, and you will increase your consistency while becoming more deliberate. Somewhere between your obligations and escape fantasies, there are tangible and worthwhile aims that are good for you and those around you. Some of the things you want may be "out there," but the way to get them is in you. It's about meaning. The more meaning, the easier to get clear. The more clear, the more focus. The more focus, the more intention. The more intention, the more intensity. Did I just oversimplify things just now? Yes. Of course, there is nuance and inherent complexity in life. However, we know that if a thing is important enough (to you), it will get done. You go to work day-in and day-out because it's directly related to your survival, albeit not in a hunter-gatherer sense. You fill up your tank or ignore the gas light, to make it on time. It's really those things you know are important, but are unclear on or have lack of belief in, that you find yourself not doing.

A chart/worksheet will pop up throughout this section to illustrate each step discussed in the process that follows. This chart/worksheet will also allow you to reverse engineer your future success. Feel free to use this on a macro level, such as planning a year or quarter, or on a micro level, such getting ready for an event or planning the week/day. It's time to step up.

Wants - Your top step

What do you want? By now, you may be sick of me asking this question. I love this question. It kind of burrows in the more you hear it, ask it, and work to find the answer. It can expose your opacity. It can expose the BS you might tell yourself and others.

Asked enough times, aside from you wanting to punch me in the face, it is THE question. It almost starts to beg, "Why am I here?" Almost, but not quite. It's like the cousin of "Why am I here?" As we all know, cousins are like the brothers and sisters we wish we had!

So going into a year, quarter, week, or single event, you want to look at the question, "What do you want?" in this way: How easy will my head rest? How triumphant will I feel / be—once I get, achieve, or do what I want? For this intervention, what I want is for you to tap into your true desire.

THE WANT

What do I want?

Goals - Get on another level

Your wants, if they are really coming from your heart and mind (AKA your gut), are the highest aim. Most of us have goals. Life goals. Relationship goals. Career goals. Really though, those goals are our wants. I know I am splitting hairs, but here is how it shakes out:

- The soccer team wants to win. In order to win, they must score more GOALS than the other team.

- The football team wants to win. In order to win, it sometimes comes down to one field GOAL!

- The basketball team wants to win. The team that wins scores the most... You got it—GOALS.

This is why the things you want are not your goals. The want is bigger than the goal(s). They may be achievable and definitely aspirational, but are they operational? Your goals literally help you Get On Another Level! Hitting your goals puts you in a place above where you were.

**Coachable Moment:

The reason many people don't get what they want—in a big way at least—is not due to lack of ability. It is due to the fact that they don't see how to get from where they are now to their highest aim. The distance is too far, and there is no path to get there. No goals. They mistake what they want for goals.

So, If you want to stay in the game, play your best game, and be consistent about it, you (and your brain) will need to see some movement along the way. Seeing progress is a great incentive to keep going. Otherwise, it's easy to talk yourself into the merits of mediocrity.

The job right here, right now, is to take those things you want and distill them down into bite-size chunks. How many points do you need to put on the board to get what you want? You want to double your sales in a year? What goals would help you get there? You want to run a marathon next year? How much do you run (or walk) now? How fast is your 5k? How many miles a week would prepare you to compete in that marathon? You want to be closer with your children or spouse? How much time a week can you devote to them, uninterrupted? What experiences can you create in the next three months? You want to make next week the best week ever? What are the goals that need to be met to allow for that to happen?

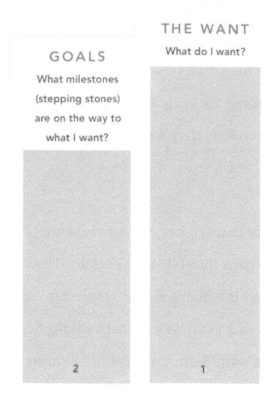

THE WANT

What do I want?

GOALS

What milestones
(stepping stones)
are on the way to
what I want?

2

1

Expectations. They're not what you'd normally expect.

Achieving your goals is all about expectations. Expectations are the things you can do that are within 80-90% (<— Totally not a scientific number, but holds true!) in your control that will move you closer to your goals. Most make the mistake of expecting to win, or not expecting to win, and that is a problem. Why? The outcome is based on a lot of external circumstances. It's too uncertain and out of your control. Simply put, you can't guarantee to win because you haven't done enough to get there. You haven't won yet! In Las Vegas the house always wins. Sure, some people "hit it big" at the tables or slots, but we know betting is entertainment and gambling can become a serious problem. Don't be the vacationer looking to get lucky. Be the serious investor looking to build wealth (and wellness).

**Coachable moment:

In the spirit of brutal honesty, the rich do get richer. It's a compound-interest-math-kind-of-thing. It's also a bit about the company they keep once a threshold is crossed—income-wise, skills-wise, or otherwise. Which is why the money is made before the trading happens. Those who do well in the market have an investment plan inclusive of an exit strategy. That plan most likely has thresholds that guide certain behavior. Once you reach a certain threshold of education, your peers and opportunities generally increase. Once you reach a threshold in performance (work or sports), your opportunities multiply. Once you reach a threshold of income, the effort to manage your wealth can be greater than it was to make—from a stress standpoint, at least.

When you look at what you want, it's generally external. Something outside of you. When you look at your goals, those are generally external — the milestones you need to meet in order to get what you want. When you look at your expectations, I want you to go internal. Expecting to win is fine. Expecting to hit your goals is fine. However, if you are expecting the former and latter without any expectation of what you can do to get there, then inconsistency will ensue at best. Your expectations have everything to do with what you are prepared to do and what you can do in order to reach the goals on the way to what you want. Skilled investors control their behavior when building a strong portfolio. Your expectations don't guarantee the win, but they can certainly get you closer to achieving the goals that will help you to the win. What do you expect of yourself? What can you do today with certainty — this week, this month — that will allow you to reach your goals?

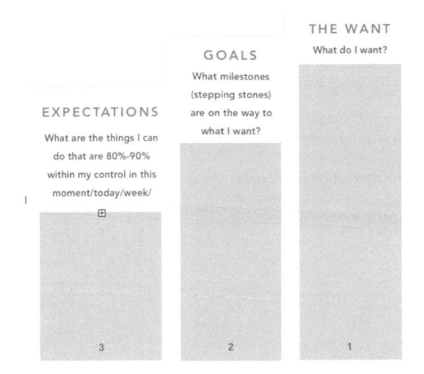

THE WANT

What do I want?

GOALS

What milestones
(stepping stones)
are on the way to
what I want?

EXPECTATIONS

What are the things I can
do that are 80%-90%
within my control in this
moment/today/week/

3   2   1

Focus. The bottom step

The bottom step, or the first step to meeting your expectations is FOCUS. What are one, maybe two things you can focus on that would allow you to meet your expectations, per the model provided in this book? It's pretty simple, but it can also be the most difficult to flesh out. For some it's a word. For others it's a behavior. I suggest you take your list of expectations and pick out one or two things that resonate with you most. Chances are there is a word, or action (maybe both) that hit you in your feels. Pick that thing—or two—that will compel you to meet your expectations. Write it down. The best of what you can get out there is based on what you have in your heart and mind. Internal consistency leads to external consistency. What drives you, drives you. Step Up!

Focus — > Expectations — >Goals ->Wants.

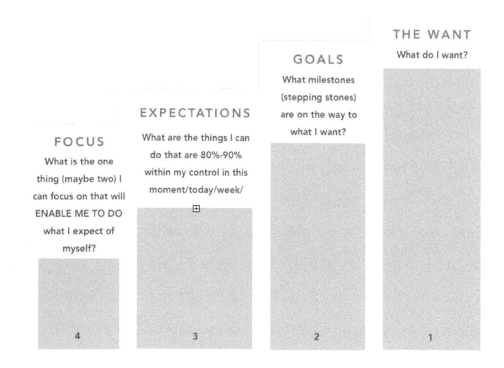

THE WANT
What do I want?

GOALS
What milestones (stepping stones) are on the way to what I want?

EXPECTATIONS
What are the things I can do that are 80%-90% within my control in this moment/today/week/

FOCUS
What is the one thing (maybe two) I can focus on that will ENABLE ME TO DO what I expect of myself?

4   3   2   1

10

Oh, You HAVE the Energy!

Energy takers - complicating, complaining, comparing, & worrying.

Complicating

The reason we tend to overcomplicate things when a project is important or big is because we have somehow deduced that it has to be complicated in order to achieve the important or big thing. Here's the dirty little secret about making things complicated: You have a great excuse as to why you fell short. It was just SO big and complicated!

In all fairness, some things ARE inherently complicated. Shorting the housing market back in 2007/2008 *was* a complicated trade. Explaining why you and I receive and generate different social media algorithms *is* complicated. You as an individual *are* complex—mixed emotions, contradictory behavior (and beliefs). We have thoughts and feelings run through our bodies, while at the same time, our bodies maintain an overwhelming homeostasis. Complicated. Still, the premise behind these complexities are actually pretty simple.

- The 2007 "Big Short" housing trade was simple: Too many people would be upside down in their homes, and too many banks made too many risky loans. There was a tremendous upside to betting on the eventual market failure vs. everyone else betting on constant growth.

- The premise for social media algorithms is simple: keep you on the platform as long as possible with news, posts, and ads that interest you based on your tracked behavior.

- The premise for you reading this book is simple: What can you do to improve life for yourself and those with whom you are connected?

Complicated is ketogenic, paleo, macros, calorie counting, heart rate monitoring, and zone training. Simple is eating less and exercising more. Complicated is trying to control everything or everyone. Simple is you focusing on what you can control and allowing others to be who they are—not that they need your permission! Complicated is avoiding the tough, avoiding the discomfort, and avoiding what in many cases is inevitable. Simple is dealing with the tough, sitting with the discomfort, and facing what in many cases is inevitable. Simple. But not easy!

By now you probably have a personal reel of your own greatest hits and misses running through your head. If so, keep the reel running! Here's what you can do if you find yourself overcomplicating things,:

Start! Make a first step. Not *the* first step. A first step. If you are confused about which first step, pick one. You'll gain the clarity once you begin. Too many of you have already found defeat through analysis paralysis. Just go back to whatever the first step is, and start over. One foot in front of the next. I wish it were sexier, but sometimes winning looks rather ugly as it's happening. Occam's razor may not always hold up scientifically, but as a general rule of thumb, making the fewest assumptions based on the evidence available to you is definitely a good place to start. Damn, there goes that word again—start! Even your GPS works better once you start, because it cannot tell which direction you are facing or headed until you start to move!

Complaining

I know this isn't exactly a polite thing to ask, but, what happens to you when you hear other people's children whining and complaining? Heck, what happens to you when you hear your own children complaining? Or maybe your employees? Or even that friend that you try to keep at a fair distance?

We complain when we don't want to do something. We complain when we think something is unfair. We get all out-of-sorts when we lack the competency/confidence/slash/wherewithal to get that thing done. Oh, and we complain when we think something's too complicated!

Robert Sapolsky's research at Stanford University shows complaining literally shrinks an area of your brain "critical to problem solving and intelligent thought." It feels good to vent, but be careful. Complaining ultimately promotes more complaining. And when you complain, your body releases a stress hormone called cortisol. When this happens, energy is diverted to survival. Survival mode keeps you alive, but only just. Keep in mind that just staying alive is a pretty low bar outside of life-or-death situations. Survival mode short-circuits rational (or better) thought. Short-circuited thought leads to reaction rather than response. While you may be good at shooting off of your back foot, it's only a skill you want to pull out when it has to be done. Lebron is dangerous shooting off his back foot, but he is a much more formidable opponent when he is driving the lane.

So let's minimize the complaining. Your job here is to do the following things:

First, armchair quarterback the other people in your circle. Become a researcher yourself. Look for the complainers and take notes. How does their complaining affect you and others around them, physically and emotionally? How productive are these complainers? Take mental snapshots and place them in the file cabinet. Take notes as well. Please remember to code them! You really don't want anyone to know you're "observing" them, even if it's for your—and their—own good.

The next thing I want you to do is time travel. Yes, time travel! Go back to your earliest memories. What was your behavior when things were tough? Ignore the circumstances and work only to think about your behavior. Did you succeed by taking big bites, or by reducing the work into smaller chunks? If you knew then what you know now, how would you handle some of the tougher moments in your business, sport, and life? What lessons can you take from the past and apply to current situations? Complaining is a MAJOR energy killer… AND, it makes you a drag to be around. If you find yourself complaining about other people, remember you are the common denominator in all of your relationships, and you can always surround yourself with other people.

If you must complain, set a time limit for the pity party — -and maybe a complaint limit. Every good party has an end, and I would think if you were stuck at a dud of a party, you would want to get out of there quickly. Finally, get in the habit of finding the silver, gold, and platinum linings to your situations, mishaps, mistakes, and circumstances.

Comparing

Expecting to *be* as fast as Usain Bolt *is*, won't necessarily encourage you to get on the starting line. Expecting to be as investment savvy as Warren Buffet is, will only frustrate the novice, expert, or even experienced investor.

I used to go on a corporate ski trip every year. During that trip, one of the planned events was a poker night. When in town, the host of the trip had standing games with his friends and sometimes other notable figures. Legend has it that a famous actor was in town and wanted in on the game. The gentleman and his friends politely declined, saying they didn't have room. That night, the mission was truly impossible. Even the rich and famous get — and feel — left out at times! By the way, I don't really know if the story is true or not. However, given what I do know about the players and the game, I tend to think this legend is fact.

If you find yourself measuring yourself against others, make sure *you're* aligned with *your* metric. If you are training for your first marathon, don't compare yourself to Natascha Badmann, one the most successful triathletes ever. Instead, measure yourself against where you were a year ago. If you're trying to be the top sales person, don't compare yourself with the Wolf of Wall Street. Instead, compare your stats with your past best or the best in the same company and category. There are levels to your success. There are levels of success. Understand the levels.

I recognize benchmarking is important. I also know it is hard to ignore your friends, siblings, neighbors, or anyone who shares your space. But remember, they are looking at you, too! And they are not looking at you, too! So I want you always to ask yourself this: Do people who compare you to them know ALL of the relevant information about YOU when it comes to their comparisons—good and bad? No, they don't. And the same goes for your comparisons and assumptions about them. You don't have the full story either—so don't make a side-by-side comparison.

Talent and self-esteem are related, but one does not guarantee the other. Rather than comparing what you have and don't have with your neighbor, sibling, competitor, or old college roommate, I want you to focus on building your self-efficacy—your ability to execute or figure it out if you lack the skill, knowledge, or resources. Your metric ultimately comes down to you meeting your expectations. If you are falling short, what can you do to measure up? (Feel free to refer to back to the "Walking Strong" bit of this book.)

Worrying

There is no future in future telling. I would love to tell you to stop worrying. But based on personality, upbringing, values, culture, and life experiences, I will say this: Let's practice keeping that anxiety in check!

You don't control your employees; you manage them. If that,

even!

You don't control all change; you manage it.

You don't control your anxiety; you manage it.

But it's not about managing others, change, or anxiety. It's about controlling yourself.

If you are responsible to your duties as a professional, family member, or teammate, then you are responsible for managing your stress and anxiety. Most everyone has stress around something, so this probably isn't new news: Anxiety zaps you of energy and can literally make you sick. Unchecked, anxiety leverages you in the worst way:

- It robs you of reason and rationality, as well as creativity and positivity.
- It floods your body and brain with stress hormones. Not good for your brain or your physical health.
- It makes you perceive things, situations, and others as threats — or bigger threats than they are.
- Ironically, anxiety causes fatigue and ruins your sleep. How the hell can you be tired and not sleep? Anxiety, that's how!

Your job here is to do several things to help you with anxiety:

- Identify your triggers. What is the situation or circumstance? How do you react? What is your behavior? What was the result/impact/consequence of those behaviors?

- Make it a priority to take care of yourself. Eat well — or even better: Get rest, move, and get some sun (wear sunblock, of course.) Practice meditation or yoga.
- Keep a running list of things you can control and things outside of your control. Do your best to create plans around things you can control.
-

- ****If you find you are constantly worrying or that most of your worry is irrational/improbable — find the help of a trained therapist or medical professional.**
-

Everyone has different stressors, and everyone manages stress differently, but there are healthy ways of managing stress, and there are unhealthy ways of managing stress. Just like there are ways you can manage a team that can leave them feeling motivated and empowered, or bored and just going through the motions. Dig into stress management that's sustainable and generally leaves you feeling healthier and happier. In fact, create some stress around it — I mean, if you're going to be stressed anyway, why not have it work for you rather than against you?!?!

Energy givers - gratitude,acceptance, simplifying, & focusing

Gratitude Inventory

Take a gratitude inventory. Seems simple, doesn't it? Almost a little trite?

"BE grateful", "Count your blessings." It is simple, and not easy. My bet is most of us don't practice this enough. I'm not saying you aren't grateful. I am saying you probably don't practice gratefulness. There is a difference. If you think the difference is small, it is. Those who perform at the highest levels in—I don't know… everything—know it's a game of splitting hairs, looking at the fine print. Not taking talent, success, and opportunities for granted.

You might be a hard-charger with goals that require a ton of work and even more attention. And I, like you, still have things on my list to achieve. But here's the thing: As you move toward a goal, you experience dissonance, the obvious awareness that you aren't where you want to be, and that doesn't even take into account the learning curve, dealing with new problems, finding new solutions, on and on and on. That dissonance can cause discomfort, anxiety, unease — possibly even disease.

Meanwhile, you are hard on yourself emotionally by thinking you are a failure or you're somehow not measuring up. All of this while you're most likely sitting in the midst of the results of your previous successes! It could be that some of you are now in a place you wanted be just a few years, months, weeks ago. Yet here you are, looking for the next thing. What we forget is where we are now, and what we have now, may have been what we wanted just a few years, or months prior. You are, in fact, here! So recognize that being where you are now *is* a mark of success, whether you survived or thrived! This might be obvious, but if you're here, isn't that proof you have gotten through everything you've been through?

What I am asking you to do is to look up. I know you have been told to put your head down and go to work. I want you to take the time to look up. What do you see? Are your surroundings pleasant? Are you in a climate controlled room? Do you have a window nearby? How expensive is your watch, or the phone in your pocket? Do you love someone? Does someone love you? What about the things that have you stressed? Could you have imagined worrying about these things one year, five years, ten years prior? If you answer honestly, I would bet many of you are already sitting in the box seats of life. You are allowed to celebrate where you are AND work toward where you want to go next. It doesn't have to be either/or. So practice looking up. Practice acknowledging the things you do have—big, little, or in between. It will help fuel you to achieve. Both your brain and your heart will be better for it.

Acceptance

You may not be where you want to be. But, if you deny it, excuse it, or are unwilling to break your circumstances down into acceptable units of facts, it'll be very difficult to move past the obstacles that present themselves in a career or lifetime. Learning to practice radical acceptance will refine your tolerances for what is and isn't acceptable as you take on the challenge of living up to your vision of a good life. To get there, you'll need a system to take inventory and categorize you, your life, and how you are performing.

To make things simple, answer the following questions with a simple yes or no:

Am I happy (or good) with where I am in my Business / Work?

Am I happy (or good) with where I am in my Health / Sport?

Am I happy (or good) with where I am in my Life / Relationships & Experiences?

Am I not okay with where I am in my Business / Work?

Am I not okay with where I am in my Health / Sport?

Am I not okay with where I am in my Life / Relationships / Experiences?

Now, break it down even further. How did you arrive at those answers?

Before you go waxing poetic or defending yourself, remember, to ERR (E-R-R) is human:

E: What were the EVENTs that led up to your current state in your business, sport, and life?

R: What were your RESPONSES (or REACTIONS) to those events?

R: What are your RESULTS based on those actions? (You should already have a good idea of this if you answered the questions honestly about being good or not with where you are).

Take some time to analyze your findings. What are the patterns (behaviorally or situationally) that keep coming up? How about timing? Too soon, too late, not enough time? That's a big one when things come down to the wire! Once you see the ugly—the stuff you just listed and analyzed—the ugly is more easily avoided.

By "see" I mean really see, not just notice. Can you stand to look at your own train wrecks? If so, your brain has literally just started a self-correcting process. Just because your brain is self-correcting, doesn't excuse you from being proactive.

Repair your past. Though events already happened, chances are good that some patterns keep presenting and repeating. The way to fix this is… to fix this. Take your past events, cringeworthy moments, biggest fails, and write down what you would do differently — other approaches and perspectives you could have taken. From there — because this is not a game of would have, could have, should have! — write down your fixes in the present or future tense. In other words, get rid of the would, could, and should in your fixes. "I could've been more patient," is weak. "I will sleep on it and make a decision tomorrow," is gangsta. "I should try to go to the gym more often" is soft. "I'm committed to training three times a week and tracking my progress," is pro!

Once you have your fixes written down, internalize it. Meditate on it. Apply it as soon as possible. This will be harder than you think. I suggest asking someone to hold you accountable to these changes in your behavior. This means showing some vulnerability with someone you can trust. You know history repeats itself. But you don't have to repeat history! Learn to do versions of this regularly. Take inventory of where you are. Radically and unflinchingly accept that you are here now, then start to make the necessary shifts to move in your chosen direction.

Focus

How many things can you do at once? Plenty! If you do things deliberately and intentionally—and—not at once! Focus is the antidote to worry. Not that it will keep you from worrying, but being focused on the want, goals, expectations—the tasks at hand—will keep you moving productively despite your worry!

Here are a four techniques that you can use when you need to focus your mind:

1. Make sure those calories have nutrients! Rather than think, "How much can I do?" Think: "How effective do I want to be?" Think: "How effective can I be?"

You want to start preferring being productive over being busy. Food is a great example to illustrate this concept. We all eat! Five hundred calories is 500 calories. But, 500 calories of potato chips, soda, and a processed microwave lunch is NOT the same as 500 calories of healthy greens, whole grains, and grass-fed whatever. The junk may fill your stomach, but it doesn't fill the void. You don't need junk calories, nor do you need busy work! Busy being productive differs from busy being busy. If you find yourself busy with very little efficiency or productivity, well, that's futility. Don't you think?

2. Talk yourself into winning! Set an intention for the day, and let that be your mantra. Tell yourself.   "I am doing this."

"This is happening"

"I'd rather do it now"

"I might as well do X... "

"I will check on (whatever's currently distracting me) later!"

This tactic, admittedly not sexy, somewhat clichéd, and parodied on late-night sketch comedy, is surprisingly effective and habit-forming! Say it, repeat it, talk yourself into focus.

**Coachable Moment:

I can appreciate how you might feel stupid talking to yourself, but you are always talking to yourself. Not taking the time to talk yourself into winning because you might feel stupid is a great example of protecting your ego, rather than allowing yourself to be happy. (Refer to Essential Questions)

3. Increase your awareness. Paradoxical, yes, but if you've ever been in a flow state or "the zone" — in sports or otherwise — I bet it would be filled with specifics and details related to that slice of time while in the flow. Practice hyperawareness of yourself, your feelings, your strengths, your weak spots. Work with yourself to direct your own system toward what focuses you. Breathing exercises, meditation, and yoga are great ways to find this awareness.

4. If you don't trust age-old practices backed by what most prominent experts know in neuroscience — or if your ego is in the way of you meditating, doing breath work, or yoga — then practice slowing down. In racing we would often say, "Slow down to go faster!" I like to say, "Slow down to go faster or further!" Here are some ways to slow down and stay focused:

- Fight for your set-up — own your space. This means giving yourself space between whatever you are coming out of and about to go into — home to work, work to play, task to task, etc.

- Give yourself some silence before your day begins or before you shift from one thing to the next. This may sound obvious, but limit your distractions and go dark once a day (not dark as in mood, but dark as in silent mode). Look at your schedule, pick, and stick to a time — no phone, no talking. I like throwing a ball against a wall, breathing exercises, or stretching during these times. Again, the goal here is to find ways for you to slow down so you can operate in a fast-paced world. The few seconds or minutes you take to slow down will be the extra percentage points needed as things come down the wire! Take the time to make the time.

Since we are being honest here, those energy-takers are not really takers. The energy-takers don't rob you of energy; they disincentivize you from persistence. Complaining, complicating, comparing, and worrying distract you from the work. But they are, in fact, energy. Which is why when you complain, complicate, compare, and worry — especially out loud — there is a release of some sort. Some call it catharsis. Over the past decade or so, I have been working with the supposition that while it may feel good to release negative energy, it's more important to channel it. You and your coach or therapist can work through when it's better to release vs. channel. Either way, it's energy, and you got it!

The energy-givers are the direct antidote to the takers, but they don't incentivize as much as they boost. Think of the energy-givers like mind and heart vitamins. Gratitude, acceptance, simplification, and focus help provide immunity. They build you up and keep you protected emotionally and mentally, if you choose to recognize and put them into practice. It's natural not to want bad things to happen to you. You know the feeling of overwhelm and stress. No one can guard you against life happening, despite your best efforts. Gratitude, acceptance, simplification, and focus help you realize, over time, that life doesn't happen to spite you. As important as we are, none of us are that important. If the world has conspired against you, you are probably doing something terribly right or terribly wrong! In either case, the remedy is still the same.

You may be compelled to look at someone else's life and think, "I wish I had their life."

I strongly urge you to want and wish for YOUR life!
You can be the GOAT:

Gratitude
Ownership
Action
Trust   dr.j rich

Home

"Once you realize the joke *is* on you. Neither the spotlight nor the anonymity will be a thing. "

11

Paradox and Irony Are Built In

It's only fair that it's not fair.

More, better, and happier exist, but it wouldn't have much value if less, worse, and sadder didn't. You are not brave because you are not scared. You are brave because you act despite your fear. The other is needed even though it is not wanted. People love to buy the new shoes or the shiny new part for their bike, but hate to pay the electric bill or change the flat tire. The other is wanted even though it is not needed.

Life is complicated, nuanced, and often tragic. Yet, here we all are, most of us trying to make this thing work better. It's like perpetual camping. Yes, it's rough, but for some reason, we get something out of working to make things more livable. Ironically, from a camping perspective, those seeking the most comfort tend to enjoy less and work harder, while those enjoying themselves more are comfortable with less. On a macro level, we use discrimination to fight it, and we seek equality to gain advantage—irony and paradox all in one. On a micro level, you embody the same principles, too. As much as you have grown, learned, and evolved, you are the same person—except for the fact that you have also changed. Hopefully for the better.

Here's why it's fair that it's not fair.

If everybody could do everything, nothing would be worth anything. More specifically, you have interests, talents, and gifts. Whether they are inherent or inherited, those things are yours. The person next to you is in the same boat, but most likely has different interests, talents, and gifts. Add in varied circumstances, times, cultures, places, and variables not mentioned, multiply all those factors by some huge number (I am not a math person), and there is an exponential amount of diversity as it pertains to what and how a person can provide value in the world, to the world, and for the world. The more you are developed in either your chosen area or within your talent/skillset, the more you can provide value to others who may lack, need, or want your talents and skillsets. That is your advantage. You, inevitably, will need someone else's talents and skills for things you either cannot do, or are not willing to do. From a commerce perspective, we trade on others' advantages. You might be able to build the fence, but your talent is really in coding, or science. It may not be fair that science is difficult for me, but it is fair that I can build the hell out of a fence and have all of the correct tools to do so. Someone programs the machines to build the tools or survey the land. I need those tools to build the fence so the neighbor's kids and dog don't fall into your pool. If there are areas where we overlap in interests, skills, or talent, then maybe working together will be more enjoyable, or we can grab a beer on the weekend.

Even within a given domain, using sports as an example, the talent and skillsets are similar, almost indistinguishable. However, even within the same range exists a stratification of advantages. Youth might be needed on one team, whereas experience is more valued on the other. Intellectual ability might not be of high value on some clubs, but held in high regard in others. The hope is what you have can help fill the gap, solve the problem, or complete the picture for the other. Within a team, every player brings what they have to the table to make the plays and win more games than they lose. Again, all trading on advantages. You could say exploiting those advantages.

In relationships, what brought you together just might have been the fight, the weed, the arrest, or same interests. Fate allows us to find one another, and our differences will enable us to leverage one another. And I use the word *leverage* in a good way, like leveraging the fact that your friend is a good listener just after a parent has passed, or leveraging the fact that your wife has a keen understanding of legal documents before you sign that contract for a loan. It's not fair that one sibling got all the looks and the other all the brains, but it's only fair for them to leverage their brains or looks to build something for themselves. Ironically, you wouldn't be surprised if each sibling was jealous of the other for what they perceive themselves as not having. As I said, paradox and irony are built in.

It could happen to you.

While it's beyond my pay and scope to speak on physics, quantum theory, or the fundamental laws of the universe, I suspect and observe that universalities exist across all hierarchies/structures (social, political, economic…even familial). One such observation is that we often become that which we protest. Or, to pose this as a question: Would you really act differently, once you are in the position of the other doing the acting?

I saw an old video in which then-senator Joe Biden urged President Bush not to nominate a supreme court justice due to the upcoming election. Yet, several election cycles later, the then-VP Joe Biden, and POTUS, Obama, wanted to nominate someone to the supreme court despite the imminent election (or maybe because of it?). It was precisely what Biden was urging against when Bush was in charge. This is not about making a political statement. This is about making a statement on how we all face a decision to cross that proverbial bridge when we get to it. Because of our experiences, genetics, stories, upbringings, differences, and specialties, we assume "our" situation is different than "their" situation. And it is. Until we are placed in their position.

Not to cast a black-and-white cloak over complex issues, but context does matter for sure. It is curious, though—the people who find themselves in situations where "they would've handled it differently"—often don't handle things differently. "Resist!" But only if you resist the right things. "Free speech!" Just make sure you say the right thing in the right way. "I'll never be like my parents." Oh, how lucky some of us would be if that were so. When you find yourself telling your kids, "Because I said so," you have crossed that bridge.

As a clinical psychologist, I have worked in crisis homes and day-treatment centers. What was interesting to me was not so much the clinical work. It was the stories of how some of the patients arrived at those places. Yes, the bulk of them had a rough upbringing inclusive of abuse, drug use, neglect, and lack of financial resources. However, that was not everyone's situation. A deal gone wrong. One drink too many. Jobless too long. Boom! They find themselves in a place they'd never thought they'd be. Schizophrenia doesn't usually set in for males until their late teens and early 20s, and late 20s to early 30s in women. There WAS no good reason for many of those clients to be there, but they were.

According to the National Institute of Mental Health, schizophrenia and other psychotic disorders occur at a rate of 0.25%-0.65%. So, within a given population of high-functioning

professionals (white or blue collar), "normal people" can find themselves in very abnormal circumstances.

I say this not to scare you, but to impress upon you a healthy respect for your life. Because it can happen to you, the converse of the grim realities are also true. Some of the kids who went to the day-treatment facility made it through school, found careers, and are now raising healthy families. Every day someone is making it — getting the job, securing the funding, becoming a champion, putting someone else through school. It just can't be that all of those people were born into it or had perfect starts in life. No matter what you were born with or how you came into this world, it's up to you to lose it, keep it, or grow it.

Change-thinking.

It's the last hour of the international flight that seems the longest. The last few pounds are the hardest to drop. The last days of school before graduation are very much like, "Why am I still here?" As you move closer toward the thing you want, you'll notice that you feel something from the anticipation. Excitement, impatience, relief, pressure, anxiety — it's at these moments we become both acutely aware of where we are and completely clueless of how we are doing, or vice versa. You want to be "there" or "done." That "thereness" and "doneness" also represents the end of a thing and the uncertainty of another. Losing and winning at the same time, proficiency and ineptness at the same time. This is normal. It's inherent in the game. This is how most of us are built. Keep in mind, we can also be proficient in our insecurity, doubt, or bad habits. It's a scary thing to cross over, whether it be from addiction to sobriety, graduation to career, or from good to great. Rest assured people do it all the time. While it may not be fair how you got in the preceding predicament, it's only fair that you have and can do what it takes to break into the next level. Regardless where the comma or decimal point is in the number, or what it is you want to do next, it is a big deal when you work to get there.

The reason why you can play as big as you want is because it's all made up. Somebody created the World Series, somebody (or a group of people) created the Super Bowl. Someone even created Christmas! I don't say this to diminish those things, because those things are amazing, and I love sporting events and holidays.

You, sitting at home reading this.

You, driving your car listening to this.

Wherever you may be in the world — you can make something up.

In your brain — the space between your ears — you can think something up, and it will seem to others that you pulled it out of thin air! And that thing you thought up, or welled up from your heart and guts, can become something of value that impacts people, helps people, entertains people, or changes the trajectory for you and your people.

For those of you who want to play big, here's what happens: We say we want to win (using "win" as a generic term for attaining a clearly defined result). And, we do want to win! But the conversation in our heads doesn't always allow us to speak honestly about what we want. Some of us finally get to the arena, pitch, or interview, and we shy away from not only what we want, but how great we can actually be. Our self-talk goes something like this:

"I just want to to the best I can."

"I just want to do what I know how to do."

I appreciate that. Who wants to sound like an egotistical jerk? It is noble to want to do the best you can. From a brain and performance perspective, it's definitely good to focus on what you know how to do. But, if I am being honest, part of you is scared to admit what you really want for fear of somehow jinxing it, or even worse, the thought of stating what you want out loud AND that thing not happening is too unbearable. Thus, we play this little game in our heads in the heat of the action… in the midst of going for the win. In other words, we're kind of changing the plan last minute. Now, if all you really want *is* to do your best — regardless of results — great. There are many who find peace in that. But for those of you who have a clearly defined result, if you really want the title, the person of the year award, the best grades, then don't deny it. If the win is what you're there for, then recognize there's a responsibility to that want.

The responsibility, by the way, is not the prerequisite behaviors it will take to accomplish your victory. The real responsibility is in dealing with yourself as you get closer to your win. Dealing with the stress. Dealing with the fact that you may be on pins and needles until it happens. The fact that it may not be as fun, or as easy, or as painless, as you thought. It might feel like you're suffocating until that last moment. It's facing the fact that, for as far as you can tell, you can't bear to think about not winning because that would be another source of stress and blow to your emotional state, given what you want to accomplish. There may come a point where your brain and your heart will do everything it can between now and the final seconds to tell you it's okay if *IT* doesn't happen. And this is the real kick in the pants. You probably will be okay if it doesn't happen! But in your heart of hearts, can you stand to come up short again? Especially, when you've stated — at least to yourself — just how far you want to go?

————

Pause.

Breathe... in through the nose and out through the mouth.

————

At this point, we not only want to be clear, but very grown-up about what's at stake for you. Your wins. Your wants. Your life. "Living your best life" may be a meme to some, but if you can define what that means, I'm willing to wager there are clear ways to measure if it is actually happening as it's happening. If you really want to be a World Champion, honor that. If you really want to create cures for illnesses, honor that. If you really want to provide for your family, honor that. We're all prize fighters to some degree. In the world of boxing or MMA, the closer a fighter gets to the championship fight, the harder the opponents he will face. Once in the championship bout, that fighter has every opportunity to quit. We discussed that earlier. But, if the fighter is there to win, then they are going to be taking some hits. If the fighter has a good team in their corner, they'll have studied the opponent, the situation, possible scenarios, and created a plan. The disciplined fighter will stick to the plan, honoring his responsibility. The fighter might be tired, stressed, or not as well-rested as he hoped. It's not that these things are okay, or even healthy, it's that the fighter is okay carrying the weight.

We won't be asked to step up to that level everyday. The example of an athlete or fighter is extreme. I use it to illustrate how we shy away from our potential and how we can talk ourselves out of winning at any level. You may not be vying for an Olympic medal or heavyweight championship. That doesn't mean you don't have your version of triumph. If you are internalizing More, Better, and Happier, what is your clearly defined win as it relates to the three domains—the one field of play?

Everyone doesn't get the call to get in the ring or be part of an Olympic team. All of us will be called up at some point for something in our lives:

"Hey, I need you to run the meeting."

"We need you to pay for the funeral."

Do you mind giving the opening remarks at the conference?"

"Our starter is injured. You're our best shot now."

"You're the only one he can turn to."

It's a question of readiness. I want you to be ready! I want you to understand that you can carry the weight and take the hits. That readiness, in many cases, is a choice. A choice to trust yourself, your abilities, and in some instances, who you are or who you can become if you are not yet "that person." That's digging deep. Much of the stress we experience in high-pressure situations is due to our unwillingness (or lack of ability) to dig. Ya' dig? Stress is not what kills. It's the perception of stress that kills. What kills performance is valuing your comfort over the responsibility to what you want. That choice about being ready? That involves a change in thinking.

You can bridge most any gap, when you offer real things of real value. At the end of the day, you may just be the most important resource you have. You can learn to code like Lovelace or Zuckerberg. You can learn to throw like Namath or Manning. You can learn most any skill from anyone. But you will never truly be like those people. You may have their fundamentals, yet fundamentally, what you bring to what you learn is why you will get the opportunity. Why you'll get a shot — provided you can stick to the plan. Provided you are willing to take some hits. In order for you to deliver or play on another level, it will begin with you changing how you think about you. Can you do more? Can you be more? Can you deliver more? Yes. Yes. And yes. If you are ready. The difference now is that if any of the answers to those three questions are "no," then it's a conscious decision at this point. I'll let you sit with that. We all have our limits.

Speaking of limits, I appreciate you allowing me to push yours. Hopefully, you've stopped, thought, fought back, resisted, agreed, or took note. As a psychologist, many of my peers talk a big game about setting boundaries. Creating limits as a way to keep oneself protected emotionally, psychologically, and physically. I don't mean to be flippant about this because it's a valuable skill. What isn't often talked about when it comes to therapy is how a skilled therapist helps the client grow and expand. It could be that for some, it takes some pushing to get the person to create healthy boundaries. In actuality, the fighter (or athlete) in my example(s) above, are rewarded for pushing their limits. That is what training is about—imposing a demand, load, or stress to promote adaptation, tolerance, and strength. Pushing limits teaches you about yourself, and it also helps you to change your thinking about what is possible. Because you experience yourself becoming more by doing more—adapting, tolerating, getting stronger—you become better. Something you thought impossible can be within your reach because you pushed and kept pushing. Now your boundaries have expanded.

Perhaps the hardest push will be to change how you think about others. Without rehashing the *Domestic Silence* chapter, let's just say we have every reason to stand behind the lines we have drawn (or have been drawn for us) in the sand. Most of those reasons are based on of a faulty premise, incomplete information, or loyalty to your preferred in-group. We all do it. Partly out of design, but also partly out of choice, and partly out of reflex.

It's the choice and reflex I am asking you to reconsider and interrupt:

"They" may not be against you as much as they are for them.

"They" are not here to make you suffer... necessarily.

"They" are not waiting to see you fail. (If they are waiting to see you fail, then you just got a gift because "they" are not needed in your life.)

"They" too, are trying to make it through their day.

Everyone on welfare does not have their hand out.

Everyone IS on some type of welfare. From food stamps to corporate tax breaks, we're all getting some help.

Millennials actually know they don't always get a trophy. And, it's a good thing they want their life to be more than just a career.

Not everyone older than you is a Boomer. And, that Boomer (who is most likely Gen-X) IS trying to do the right thing.

You're designed to spot differences. Sesame Street taught many of us to do so! *"One of these things is not like the others..."* Not all anomalies are threats. Those who disagree with you are not necessarily the opposite of you. If "people suck," then you suck. If "people are stupid," then you are, too! If you find yourself talking (thinking) like this and placing yourself outside of the term "people"—the joke is on you. In either scenario this thinking doesn't make you happier. It leads to resentment and pessimism. In both scenarios, it's most likely the case that people are not as stupid and do not suck as much as you might think—they just do stupid and sucky things. Or, you are the person doing the stupid, sucky things and just don't realize it at the time. Unless of course, you are not "people." Pragmatically, people are smart enough, despite a lack of specific knowledge or awareness about various topics and all of us take for granted our specific knowledge for general knowledge.

This is not an exercise in walking around the world like a

naive toddler. There are malevolent, narcissistic, and dumb people in the world. Those are the anomalies, not the rule! Additionally, it's most likely the case that those who act with malevolence and narcissism are doing so from your perspective, not theirs. Meaning, decent and good people do bad things, too. Extending yourself to the possibility that there is more to the other person than what you first thought, or better than what you give them credit for, will ulti-mately — over time — allow you to be happier for yourself and others. Keep your eyes open. And remember to open your mind and heart just as well.

Did you know:
Many successful people
don't feel (or think) they
are that successful?

Did you also know:
You don't have to be
extraordinary to live an
extraordinary life?

12

Restarted

More, Better, Happier is a book I've always wanted to write. As with many ideas—it is just that, an idea. A concept that sounded great in my head, but the words were hard to find when I started. Typically, my process is to take a big idea and break it down into smaller concepts in a notebook—pencil to paper. From there, those concepts become chapters, and each chapter becomes an essay or paper, more or less. I then arrange the subtitles, headings, and chapters in a way that I think makes sense for the reader.

When the words for MBH started to find their way on to the

screen, I became excited. I envisioned future early mornings and late nights of keyboarding the chapters that would eventually become my next book. However, as the words started to land on the screen, something happened that I wasn't ready for at the time. My tone was dark, and I sounded jaded. The mood was uncharacteristically ominous—and that's not me! Or was it what I had become? I couldn't escape the fact that I had the thoughts, wrote the words, and at the time, thought that I agreed with them. So, this very unfinished and barely-started book sat like many big ideas do—on a shelf in an "I'll get to it one day" pile.

I could blame it on my dad having cancer. I could blame it on my fear of not measuring up as a parent and husband. I could blame it on the dollars that weren't getting deposited. I could blame it on my wife's (healthy) skepticism about my big ideas. I wanted to blame all of those things. Regardless of whether I blamed my circumstances or not, I damn sure started to resent them. I wasn't okay with how things were going. My dad was dying. I was tired of asking my wife to bear with another big idea, and my kids needed me in a better way than I was showing up. That's why the words were dark, and that's why this book sat on the shelf.

Meanwhile, I needed me to show up in a way that I believed I could. I was raised better, taught better, trained better, and educated better. I often found myself asking, "What am I doing?" on an almost daily basis. The resentment was becoming anger. That anger was ultimately grounded in fear. And the fear was robbing me of strength. I fully believed in the MBH concept (now a premise and framework, as you have discovered), but I was growing impatient even with my own process. I was forcing myself to put out a product, trying to appeal to the right niche, and pushing to make an ever-changing arbitrary deadline. I was either forcing or stalling the process while intermittently listening to the "experts" telling me what I "should or shouldn't" do in the digital landscape of online-tech-entrepreneur-funnel-10x-pick-your-buzzword blah, blah, blah.

The math was simple, and I was on the wrong side of the equation. I hadn't factored in the equation that there was a shift happening in the world, with my family, and in me. I *was* on my way, just not there yet. It wasn't time for me to say what you've read, because I was neither ready nor positioned to say such things. It had to unfold how it did.

People often confuse how they feel with their fate. Present bias tells us how it is now is how it will be. I'm an energetic, optimistic, and mostly trusting person who was experiencing sadness and anger — not the other way around. Given this context, it's essential to acknowledge that anger need not serve as the source for MBH, but you have to know that anger, fear, and sadness might have informed the content at times. That's okay. A rich life worth living is one filled with the complete spectrum of experiences. Why was I angry? Why was I sad? The answer was not because life is unfair, or that I am not good enough. The answer is because there are people and things in my life that I love. When I realized this was the source from which I operate, the words found themselves hitting the screen.

The people closest to me owe me nothing. I, however, am indebted to you all:

My wife needs to know that I sometimes really don't know how I pulled it off, getting her to marry and stay married to me thus far. Her grace, support, and push-back is the conscience I seem to lack at times. I am fortunate to have her example.

Kids, you need to know I am undercover impressed with or proud of some of the things you do that piss me off. It's just a matter of age, time, and a bit of growth on both of our parts that you'll find your ways. Hopefully I'll have the courage to let you go as you journey outward. As for the respective ages you are now, I can't let you get away with all of it—you both know what Im talking about! I expect you to be better than me, and while that seems like a raw deal, it really isn't because I wouldn't be under-cover proud/impressed by your shenanigans if I didn't believe you both are already on your way. And... there are many ways to be better than me. Ask mom if you feel your list is too short.

To be clear — and so you can't say you haven't been told — talent (though it's nice to have), passion (though it helps you stay in the game), and looks/likes are not enough! It's easy to be comfortable. It's easy to feel guilt because you've been blessed with certain gifts, talents, and dare I say, birthright. Your starts, however, will not guarantee your finishes. It'll be up to you fall back, maintain, or improve. Fortunes can be squandered, riches can be had. Depending on when and how you actually read the previous pages (if at all!), you will understand it's not money alone that I'm referencing. Heavy stuff, I know, but I wouldn't put this to you guys if I didn't think you're capable of lifting the weight — and it will be heavy at times. I believe you both to be stronger than you think. Know that others in your life will help lift you, especially when you've shown your own effort and willingness. If you find or feel that you are lifting all the weight by yourself, remember it's because you can.

This book is my letter to you both. Trust me — it will come back to haunt you, like the lessons my father passed to me. Unlike me, Papa was a man of few words—one of the ways I improved (albeit, a debatable improvement) on our name. What I appreciated most from him was that he always did what he thought was right. You will learn, or maybe you already know, that's a lot easier said than done. The last lesson I learned because of him was that I can carry the torch (and weight) myself. I no longer need him to stand on my own two feet, even though I stood on his shoulders for so long. My jumping-off point might be considered unfair, but I don't apologize for it. It was up to me to take advantage of the privileges afforded to me, both inherent and given. It is up to you to do the same. My hope is you honor your jumping-off points by taking advantage of your gifts and talents, both inherent and given. Lastly, make sure you appreciate and share those advantages because none of them are guaranteed.

Long before I started this book, a good friend told me that I walk strongly. I didn't know what to make of his statement, but his words have always stayed with me. I think he saw in me what I almost lost sight of. I believe what he saw in me were the things I learned from my dad and the things I work to instill in you. Your More, your Better, and your Happier are not just "out there!" It's never been a destination. It has always been a way to guide you and a place that can exist within you. It's on you to decide if want that responsibility. I fully believe that both of you are up to the task. Thank you for being here,

j

13

Last Question

I know some of you skipped ahead!

How many times did you win before you got your first win?

If you were to attend a talk of mine, I would weave my election story from eighth grade into my presentation. I place part of the story — the posters, the speech, the vote — strategically in the talk as a pattern interruption and a refocus for the group. What I mention at the end of the talk — and what I left out at the beginning of this book — is that Facebook (or Meta... No ego in that company?!?!) and the other social media channels allow everyone to keep tabs on everyone, especially our old classmates. (Keep in mind I am on stage, in front of a reasonably-sized group). The story continues with the fact that of all the kids in that eighth-grade class, there is only one pro athlete, one world champion, one author, one person here talking to you right now. The crowd usually sees the tie-in, and it is a good story. There's a bit of funny, a bit of authenticity, and a bit of a happy ending sprinkled with a dash of hope on top of the bigger points about mindset, belief, and action — or resilience — depending on the talk.

All of the above is part of the reason why I placed that story in this book. The other reason is this: It's not a story about triumph, belief, or resilience. It is the story of my life, a foreshadowing into the fact that there were many times in my life where I was, and will continue to be, the only vote for myself. It's not because I am special or see what others don't. I doubt If I were to run for any office, my chances of winning have improved. But the continued casting of the ballot, in my estimation, is where I see value.

Everything about that election story holds true for all of us to some degree. There are times when you were misled. There were times when you were alone, or felt that way. There were times when things did not work out as you hoped or planned. These are inflection points. Times to decide if you want to quit, stick, or shift. Times to decide if you want your worst fears to do the talking (and they are always talking to some degree), or if you want to work on and build a stronger voice. One that keeps you moving forward. We already went through reasons why you may not be getting what you want. You are allowed to be not good enough. You decide if that is good enough or not enough for you. You are allowed to quit. You decide if you can handle the possibility of letting that opportunity or dream go. You are allowed to work hard, slow, smart, or not at all. You decide if those timelines and standards are sustainable, for you.

All the while, you live in a world with people in it. Occasionally, we bump into one another. There are markets and market conditions, trends, personal preferences, and tastes. (Using the term "markets" loosely, here. Not just referencing commerce.) Your vote for yourself and what you're doing does not mean it will be accepted, wanted, or warranted. Again, another inflection point. You get to decide what you need to learn and communicate your vision, plan, and idea better.

As you know, my first win was clearly NOT my eighth-grade election. As you also know, I am still here — and no longer back there. Yet, still playing! All of us win and lose from time to time. Are your wins and losses terminal or educational? If terminal, well then, game over. If educational, game on! If transformational, then game won! You decide.

Before you go further…

Pause.

Breathe… in through the nose and out through the mouth. Now, GO!